diet
&fitness
JOURNAL
your personal guide
to optimum health

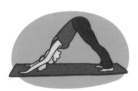

Written by Claudine Gandolfi

Illustrated by Kerren Barbas Steckler

PETER PAUPER PRESS, INC.
WHITE PLAINS, NEW YORK

Thank you to Jennifer Vagios, MS, RD, for countless hours of listening as well as counseling me; Karen Babaganov, C.H.H.C., Nutritional and Lifestyle Coach; Chris Kehoe, Personal Trainer, B.S., C.F.T.; & Stacey Wall, Personal Trainer, B.S., C.P.T., for the training and motivation provided at Fitness Together, Scarsdale, NY; and most of all to my meeting leader, Terry LaManna, from the Scarsdale & Yonkers, NY, Weight Watchers. You kept me interested in coming to the meetings and sticking with the program because of your upbeat attitude and sense of humor. I couldn't have done the monster-size portion of what I did without you.

Designed by Rebecca Lown and David Cole Wheeler

Illustrations copyright © 2018 Kerren Barbas Steckler

Visit us at www.peterpauper.com

diet
&fitness
JOURNAL

your personal guide
to optimum health

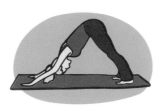

CONTENTS

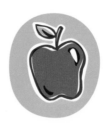

INTRODUCTION

Put down that Venti Mocha-frappa-cappa-whatzit. Banish those soft, gooey chocolate chip cookies. Say good-bye to the extra-crispy fried chicken forever. **Wait! Wait! Don't put this journal down! We're kidding about giving up the things you love!** Sure, there are things to avoid for better health, but there's really nothing you need to give up forever. You'll find a way to work in your favorites. It all boils down to choices. It's time to eat more vegetables, fruits, whole grains, complex carbs, and lean protein; they're best for your body. But, hey, you've got to feed your soul every once in a while, too. Balance is everything.

You've a valuable tool in your hands that will help you in your quest to get fit or stay fit. Studies show that recording what we eat and how we exercise helps us lose up to 50% more weight, keeps us "honest" about our diets, keeps us on track, and helps achieve our goals. It's simple: If you don't know what you're doing wrong, how can you correct it? Our *Diet & Fitness Journal* will help you target ways to improve and pinpoint weak areas and eliminate them. You may be surprised at how much you're actually putting into your mouth. But remember, you're not trying to lose "weight." You're losing fat while gaining muscle. This journal will help you do that by providing positive suggestions and a place to record your efforts. Here are a few thoughts to get you started:

- The science behind nutrition changes daily; keep your eyes on the news for updates and reversals.

- Everybody is different. You may have a different reaction to a food than a friend does. It all depends on genes and environment. Listen to your body. This journal will help you do just that.

- You cannot eat too many vegetables. Load up on the green leafy kind and the orange and red ones. Leave white veggies, especially potatoes, for rare occasions. Colorful veggies fill you up with nutrients and fiber. No one ever got fat going to town on spinach.

- You'll enjoy some fruit every day, too.
- Switch from highly processed, quickly digested carbs to complex carbs in whole grains.
- Go for lean proteins in grains, fish, fat-free dairy, eggs, poultry, and lean meat. Drink enough water to keep you hydrated.
- Take a multivitamin each day. Note: Several vitamins are fat-soluble—you'll need fat in your diet in order to absorb them.
- MOVE. Then move some more.
- Think about what you're putting into your body before you eat.
- Chew your food at least 20 to 30 times before you swallow.

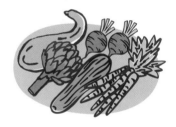

USING THE *DIET & FITNESS JOURNAL*

Using this journal is easy. It's divided into sections:

1. Information about diet, nutrition, and fitness

2. Journal pages in which to log your daily food intake and energy expenditure from activity

3. Weekly progress pages with extra tips and motivators

4. A calorie and nutrition chart for common foods. Note: In this journal, the terms "calorie" and "kilocalorie" are synonymous.

5. A "keep-motivated" personal progress chart at the back.

Try to be as complete as possible when recording your food intake and your exercise/activity. If you bite it, then write it, no matter how small!

daily food log

In the Food Log *(opposite)*, you'll record:

Day/Date/Week number

Time—*when* you eat each meal and snack, not how long it takes

What you eat, portions of food, calories, nutritional information, and anything else you want to keep track of—like Weight Watchers™ member points, or sugar content if you're diabetic and watching insulin.

Calories consumed each day (add up your daily totals)

Daily targets for calories *(to determine, see pages 28–29)*, and the percentage or grams of each type of food. Tally/record your actual percentage or grams for each.

Daily servings of water, fruits, and vegetables.

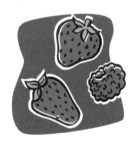

FOOD LOG

Day 5   **Date** 8/20   **Week #** 3

	Portion	Calories (kcal)	Fat (g)	Saturated Fat (g)	Sodium (mg)	Carbs (g)	Fiber (g)	Protein (g)	Other
BREAKFAST Time: 7:30									
egg whites	1/2 c	60	0	0	202	0	0	2	
feta cheese	1 oz	75	6	4	316	1	0	4	
spinach	1/2 c	4	0	0	12	0	0	0	
Breakfast Totals →		139	6	4	530	1	0	16	
SNACK Time: 10:00									
apple, gala	8 oz	131	0	0	0	34	5	1	
tea, green	8 oz	2	0	0	3	0	0	0	
Snack Totals →		133	0	0	3	34	5	1	
LUNCH Time: 1:30									
romaine	6 leaves	6	0	0	3	1	0	0	
grilled chicken	4 oz	171	3	1	59	0	0	35	
grape tomatoes	3 oz	30	0	0	0	6	1	1	
vinaigrette	2 tbs	70	5	0	129	7	0	0	
Lunch Totals →		277	8	1	191	14	1	36	
SNACK Time: 3:00									
Greek yogurt, FF	1/2 c	38	0	0	23	2	0	7	
blueberries	1/2 c	42	0	0	1	21	3	1	
Snack Totals →		80	0	0	24	23	3	8	
DINNER Time: 6:00									
skirt steak	3 oz	174	9	3	65	0	0	23	
baked sweet potato	1	103	0	0	41	24	4	2	
steamed broccoli	1 c	54	0	0	64	12	6	4	
Dinner Totals →		331	9	3	170	36	10	29	
SNACK Time: 8:00									
Blueberry muffin	1	259	13	2	208	33	1	3	
Snack Totals →		259	13	2	208	33	1	3	
Daily Totals →		1,219	36	10	1,126	141	20	93	

DAILY FOOD GOALS

target	actual	
1200	1219	calories
270	93×4	protein (g)
660	141×4	carbs (g)
333	36×9	fat (g)

water (8 oz glasses)

X	X	X	X	X	X	X	X

fruits + vegetables (servings)

X	X	X	X	X	X		

daily fitness log

In the Fitness Log *(opposite)*, you'll record:

Cardio and other workouts (aerobics, yoga, Pilates, running, treadmill, swimming, etc.) and physical activities (mowing the lawn, vacuuming, gardening, etc.). Include workout duration, intensity, heart rate, speed, and anything else you're tracking.

Strength training / weight lifting (weight machines, free weights, etc.), including reps and sets, muscle groups you're working that day.

Estimated calories burned for each activity; you'll use that number to calculate total calories burned for the day.

Net calories (calories consumed minus calories burned). You're aiming for the net number to be 500 calories below your BMR, or Basal Metabolic Rate (the number of calories your body requires to stay at your current weight) in order to lose 1 pound a week *(see pages 28–29)*. Subtract your BMR from your net calorie amount to get net calorie deficit for the day.

Vitamins/Supplements: daily dosage and quantity.

Mood (1 ☹ for bad, 8 ☺ for great) and energy level (1 for low, 8 for high) for the day.

Thoughts, moods, and feelings, in the Notes/Journal Section.

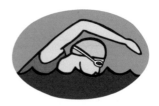

FITNESS LOG

CARDIO/OTHER	Time of Day	Heart Rate	Duration	Speed	Level	Intensity	Other	Calories (kcal) Used
elliptical	12		30	5	16			428
Calorie Totals								**428**

WEIGHTS	Time of Day	Muscle Group	Reps	Sets	Duration	Intensity	Other	Calories (kcal) Used
10 lbs.	12:30	arms	12	3	5			178
Calorie Totals								**178**

Total Calories Burned	606

Calories Consumed		Calories Used		Net Calories		BMR (Basal Metabolic Rate)		Net Calorie Deficit
1219	−	606	=	613	−	1297	=	684

Vitamins/Supplements	Dosage	Quantity
multi	1	1
vit. D	400	2
vit. C	500	1

mood

☹ 2 3 4 5 ⑥ 7 ☺

energy level

1 2 3 4 5 ⑥ 7 8

A 3,500 calorie deficit will equal 1 lb of weight loss.

Notes/Journal

woke up tired but after working out feel energized!

weekly progress section

The weekly section *(opposite)* provides ample room to record your medical statistics and measurements from week to week. Here is where you can reflect on what you've learned this week and plot strategies for next week. Do the math and discover how many pounds you should have lost (in a perfect world) in the Daily Calorie Deficit section. But don't forget—not everyone has the same kind of metabolism. You may have slower results than what you're projecting mathematically. Your body may lose this week's weight next week. Or you may have a medical condition you're unaware of; that's why it's important to check with a physician before undertaking a new fitness/wellness program.

*Fitness—if it came in a bottle, everybody
would have a great body.*

CHER

WEEKLY PROGRESS

STATS	Weight	BMI	BMR	Heart Rate	Cholesterol	Blood Sugar	Other
Last Week	190	29	1600	64		90	
Current	188	29	1595	60		90	

MEASUREMENTS	Neck	Shoulder	Chest	Waist	Hip	Thigh	Calf	Arm	Other
Last Week	13		34	42	24				
Current	12		33	41	23				

Notes/Journal

Lost two pounds this week and actually enjoyed
what I was eating + doing. Even managed to eat
out with friends on Friday.

GOALS FOR NEXT WEEK

increase cardio to 3 days a week and increase reps.
Work in that slice of pizza I was eyeing.

DAILY CALORIE DEFICIT

Day 1	200	Day 5	912
Day 2	539	Day 6	200
Day 3	456	Day 7	757
Day 4	712	Weekly Total	3,776

Waist Hip Ratio
Women <.7
Men <.9

.8

A Word About Journaling

Why does this book have places to take notes? Because most plans recommend you take stock of your feelings, frustrations, and successes and get them on paper. You may see how certain stressful days cause you to "slip" from your wellness plan.

Stressful situations cause your body to switch into "flight or fight" mode, releasing the hormone cortisol. Cortisol is wonderful—in small doses. It increases memory and immunity, and gives you a burst of energy. But after prolonged periods of stress, it makes your body store fat in your abdomen, decreases muscle tissue development, suppresses thyroid functioning, and more. If you're trying to lose weight, your job is to trick your body into giving up fat stores while building lean muscle (the opposite of what stress does).

Try to avoid situations that cause undue stress. Use proven relaxation techniques: yoga, meditation, journaling, affirmations, and naps, if you can. Recording moods and stresses can also help you identify trends like, "When I eat carbs late in the day, I feel sluggish the morning after." Recognizing such patterns will help you understand what to do. Listen to what your body is telling you.

GETTING STARTED
starting points: where we are now

First things first. Consult your doctor to make sure this program is right for you. If it is, then attach that "Before" photo and record that "Before" weight, blood pressure, resting heart rate, measurements, etc., in the "Last Week" lines of the first "Weekly Progress Log" page. Then say "bye-bye" to "Before" and "hello" to the new you!

Remember, when starting an activity or exercise program, think "baby steps." No one should run at 8 mph the first day. Instead, go for a walk. Take the stairs instead of the elevator. Stretch. Next week, do a little more: walk on an incline, try yoga, cycling, or swimming. You'll be ready for kickboxing boot camp or spin class in no time. **Note:** You'll need to change your exercise program every 4 to 6 weeks to keep it effective. Once the body gets used to certain activities, they don't have the same calorie-burning effect as they did at first. To continue your progress, change! Amp up, or do something at the same level but for a longer period of time.

There's no need for a daily weigh-in, unless you want to. Don't obsess about that scale! Body weight fluctuates naturally, based on what you've eaten, sodium consumed, how much you've exercised, the kind of exercise, and other unfathomable reasons. So, if weighing in daily, don't get discouraged by temporary "It's not working!" panic that might throw you off course.

Pay attention to what your body is telling you over longer periods of time. This isn't a race, and those who lose weight quickly tend to gain it back and then some. **Don't think of your new regimen as temporary.** Think of it as the new way you'll live longer and stronger. Love yourself.

Females, remember, you may gain up to 5 pounds during that time of month. Relax. Your metabolism fluctuates weekly (but remember, you're in this for the long haul). Don't give up.

You're the only one looking at this journal (unless you're going to share it with a doctor, trainer, or nutritionist). There's no need to "fudge" the numbers. **Be honest with yourself even on days you're not able to watch what you're eating.** Pay attention to the Nutrition Facts printed on food packages. You may be surprised at how many extra servings are contained in that tiny little packet you thought was single-serving size. Try to keep sodium, fat (especially saturated and trans fats), and sugar at a minimum.

Recent government surveys in the UK and U.S. find that more than 61% of adults are overweight, with 27% (UK) and 38% (U.S.) obese. If you're overweight, you're not alone. How did this happen? Partly because we've become sedentary, sitting at our respective desks all day instead of doing physical work, partly because we rely on pre-packaged, overly-processed food items instead of fresh produce, and partly because portion sizes have become outrageous—the food industry's promotion of "bigger is better" and "more bang for your buck" has resulted in restaurant portions that can feed four, instead of one.

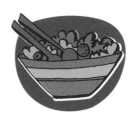

starting points: where we want to be

It's time to set goals for yourself. Want to drop 20 pounds by summer? Want to firm up and lower your blood pressure? Find out where you need to be, then set small goals. Sometimes larger goals throw us off track because they seem so, well, big. Small steps help us get there without despair.

Weight: Check out the government chart for healthy, overweight, and obese weights *(see page 30)*. These are only guidelines. Not everyone is made the same. Some people will be healthy at a higher weight than this suggests. Some may need to weigh less. Each of us is unique. Our background can predetermine our body composition through DNA. Strive to be healthy, not thin.

Blood Pressure: This should be below 120/80.

Resting Heart Rate: You should be aiming for a RHR between 60 and 80 beats per minute *(see page 31)*.

Waist to Hip Ratio: A good indicator of overall health. Body fat stored around your midsection is a risk factor for heart disease. Work to get and keep this low. To determine Waist to Hip Ratio, you'll need a tape measure. Measure your hips around the widest part of your buttocks. Then measure your waist where it's smallest, above the belly button. Divide the waist measurement by the hip measurement. Cardiovascular risk is higher for women with ratios higher than 0.85, and for men with ratios above 0.90.

THE SKINNY ON HEALTHFUL EATING
DIET is a four-letter word

The restrictions imposed by a diet can cause resistance—even other four letter words in response. So how do you trick yourself into behaving for your own benefit? **First, don't think of this as being "on a diet." You're changing the way you're eating for the rest of your life, not just for beach season.** Retrain your brain to embrace a healthy lifestyle. Those who lose weight quickly may assume "once I'm done with the diet, I can eat as much as I want." But that attitude will cause them to regain those pounds—and then some. So just go ahead and include that chocolate cake in your plan (that's what this journal is for). Then spend some extra time at the gym to make up for it. No biggie. Be accountable for what you eat, and you can enjoy the foods you love, in moderation, for the rest of your life. Nothing is off limits!

the food groups

What foods to eat? Let's look at what you'll be eating. Simply put, calories come in one of three basic forms:

- Carbohydrates (4 calories per gram)
- Proteins (4 calories per gram)
- Fats (9 calories per gram)

Again, put simply, your body feeds on carbs first, then proteins, then fats. Fad diets often promote cutting one of these from your diet. Yes, you will lose weight—you're cutting out an entire food group. But each group is essential to health.

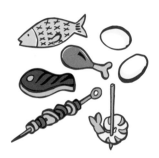

carbohydrates

Balance, and eating the right kinds of carbs, is key. Too few carbs and your brain stops functioning well. Too few carbs, and your body will make its own by depleting glucose stored in your liver. No glucose? Your liver will actually "cannibalize" it from muscle tissue. Too many carbs? Your body turns them to fat for energy storage. Blood sugar increases, more insulin is produced, possibly leading to a gradual desensitization to insulin, and the inability of your body to absorb the sugar in your blood: Type II diabetes. Not good.

About 50% of the calories you consume should come from carbs, and the complex kind should dominate your diet. So, if you're consuming 1,500 calories daily, then 750 of them (188 grams) should be from carbs. You may be thinking, "I can't possibly eat that many!" Sure you can. Carbs consist of sugars, starches, and fiber. Fruits and vegetables are excellent carb sources, and they're packed with fiber to keep your digestive tract moving and help you feel full. Keep to carbs in their most natural forms. Recommended amounts of fiber: 25–40 grams daily.

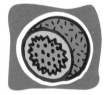

Avoid: Anything white—bleached flour, refined sugar, pasta, and rice. High fructose corn syrup is a no-no. Sweet tooth? Go for berries and fruit. Berries are high in flavonoids and other nutrients. Pomegranates, kiwi, and goji berries are super foods to incorporate into your diet. Instead of sugar, you may want to try natural sweeteners like raw honey, maple syrup, or stevia.

Chocolate? Love it! The darker, the better. Make sure it's not milk chocolate, and that it has a high concentration of raw cocoa. Flavonoids, powerful antioxidants in dark chocolate, fight cancer and heart disease, among other ailments. Who knew? Have a small piece a day (the size of one or two squares of a candy bar). No need to deprive yourself. Just don't overdo. There are still calories to count!

CARBS	
The Bad	**The Good**
Processed treats	Fresh fruits & vegetables
White flour	Whole wheat flour (NOT enriched)
Sugar, high fructose corn syrup	Agave nectar, stevia, honey
White toast	Whole wheat toast
Pasta & rice	Whole wheat pasta, brown rice
White potatoes	Yams, sweet potatoes
Milk chocolate	Dark chocolate, cocoa nibs

fats

Yep, you need 'em. Without fats, your brain won't function well. (It's over 70% fat.) You won't be able to absorb certain vitamins (A, D, E, and K). Your liver won't be able to metabolize your current fat! That's right, new fat helps burn old fat. The trick is getting the right kinds of fats. Avoid trans fats (these are fats that are solid at room temperature) and saturated fats like lard, shortening, butter, and margarine. These clog up your arteries, leading to atherosclerosis. You want unsaturated fats, specifically mono- and poly-unsaturated. These, from nuts (almonds, walnuts, pistachios), some oils (olive, safflower, canola), dark chocolate, and avocados can actually help you lose belly fat while keeping nails, skin, and liver functioning. Dairy products may have high fat content—go for low- or non-fat choices.

Fats should comprise about 10% of your daily intake of food. Again, if you're consuming 1,500 calories a day, 150 of those calories (or 17 grams) should be healthy fats.

FATS	
The Bad	**The Good**
Saturated fats, trans fats, (hydrogenated oils, margarines)	Poly- & mono-unsaturated fats (nuts, avocados, olive and canola oil)
Fried foods	Steamed, poached, grilled, raw, roasted, baked foods
Creamy dressings	Vinaigrettes
Creamy soups	Broth-based soups
Au gratin anything	Olive oil and garlic
Whole milk	Skim/fat-free milk, almond milk
Cheeses & yogurts	Low-fat or fat-free cheeses & yogurts, low-fat kefir
Premium ice cream	Slow-churned, double-churned "light" ice creams, frozen low-fat/fat-free yogurts, sorbet, sherbet

proteins

Proteins build muscle and keep skin, hair, and nails smooth and healthy. These are the building blocks of life. Don't skimp. Just like everything else, there's good protein and bad. You want to look for lean meats, not processed or fatty cuts. If you're a vegetarian, make sure you're getting protein from dairy (cottage cheese and Greek yogurt are great sources), nuts (peanut butter), beans and legumes (chickpeas, lentils), or soy (tofu, edamame); the latter three also work for vegans. Ladies, be careful about overusing soy. Plant estrogens from soy have been shown to possibly increase the incidence of women's cancers.

Protein should make up 15%–25% of your daily caloric intake. On a 1,500 calories a day plan, that would be 225–375 calories (or 57–94 grams).

PROTEINS	
The Bad	**The Good**
Hamburger	Turkey burger, veggie burger, soy burger
Fatty cuts of meat (brisket, prime rib)	Lean cuts (sirloin, London broil)
Sausage	Turkey or chicken sausage
Hot dogs	Soy dogs
Animal protein	Vegetable protein (soy, beans, nuts)

organics

Organic foods—those with a five-digit grocery store PLU# that starts with a "9"—are foods grown without the use of chemicals and pesticides. Many people believe their nutrition content is higher than that of conventional foods. If you agree, be eco-friendly and try to buy locally grown organics at farmers' markets. (Transporting organics from afar leaves a greater carbon footprint.) And make sure your purchases have a USDA "Certified Organic" seal (or EU organic logo in Europe) so you know they're not just conventional food in organic clothing.

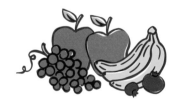

glycemic index

There's a growing trend to consider the Glycemic Index (GI), a measurement of the body's ability to process carbohydrates in foods. **Low glycemic foods keep insulin levels in balance without causing blood sugar peaks and valleys.** This helps your body stay "in tune," minimizing cravings and propensities to binge. Keeping insulin levels balanced helps you feel full, and you may be less likely to snack between meals because your energy level is up. There's an entire database of food GIs you can look up on www.glycemicindex.com. Go for foods with low GIs (<55).

when is it best to eat?

Eat when you're hungry, not because it's a certain time of day. Judge portions. Eat slowly. Put down the fork between bites. Chew your food 20–30 times before swallowing. Digestion, particularly carbohydrate digestion, starts in the mouth. If you're not chewing your food, you're not digesting it properly. The slower you eat, the less you'll eat. It takes 15 minutes for the "full" trigger to go from stomach to brain.

The most important time to eat is when you first get up in the morning. Your body has been fasting for perhaps 8 hours, and it needs nutrients to get your system and metabolism going. Keep water by your bed, and try to drink about 2 cups when you get up. Then make breakfast. Get some protein in every meal. And try to aim for 5 to 6 mini-meals of about 300 calories each (depending on your daily caloric goals) throughout the day, instead of 3 square meals and 2 snacks, as recommended in the past. By eating every 3 to 4 hours, you keep metabolism and insulin levels on an even keel. You won't experience those afternoon sugar highs and "crashes."

Working out? Eat a mini-meal of maybe 200 calories beforehand (mostly carbs, some protein). If you can eat a meal afterward, say within 40 minutes after working out, your metabolism will be at its highest peak, and you'll burn calories more quickly. Make the post-workout meal mostly protein (to help repair muscle) with some carbs.

nutrition tips & tricks

Here are some strategies to maximize your caloric burn:

- Skip the late-night snack. Going to bed a little hungry will force your body to use stored glucose, then fat, to feed its needs.
- Hungry? Drink a glass of water first. Sometimes the brain confuses thirst with hunger.
- Craving something? Wait 15 minutes before giving in. Try eating a small piece of what you're craving instead of the whole thing.
- Load that plate with vegetables. Veggies should take up half your plate, lean protein a quarter, and carbohydrates the remaining quarter.
- Use a salad plate instead of a dinner plate for your entrée. The smaller size will make portions more manageable.
- Once cooked, portion out your food and freeze leftovers in serving size containers.
- Share dessert.
- Don't eat take-out from the container. Put it on a plate to prevent overindulgence.
- Dress up the dinner table. Eat sitting down at it. Don't eat in front of the TV.
- Don't put a serving platter on the table. That only encourages everyone to take more.
- Embrace color! Red, orange, purple, as well as leafy green vegetables, are loaded with antioxidants—they're powerhouses for healthy eating.
- Try new fruits and vegetables. You may be missing out! Don't be afraid to experiment.
- Eat new grains. Instead of rice or wheat, try quinoa, spelt, or oat groats.

- Drink enough water. Some suggest dividing your weight by 2 and drinking that many ounces a day. Drink a glass of water when you get up in the morning to re-hydrate yourself from sleep.
- You don't need to "clean your plate." Stop when you're not hungry.
- Say "No, thank you" to food pushers at work, at home, and at parties. You're not responsible for others' actions—only your own.
- Start meals with soup or salad. You'll eat less of your entrée.
- Pass on the bread basket.
- Keep that sodium count low! The UK Food Standards Agency recommends no more than 2,300 mg per day, and the USDA reduced it to 1,500 mg a day for those with high blood pressure. Watch out for restaurant meals and canned and packaged goods.
- While you're watching your sodium intake, do the same for sugar. The American Heart Association recommends that women have no more than 6 teaspoons (25 g) of sugar a day, and men no more than 9 teaspoons (37.5 g). Half of this can be from added sugars, the other half from naturally occurring sugars. The English NHS's recommended limits are 50 g and 70 g for women and men, respectively.
- Your fiber intake should be between 25 and 40 g a day. Know the difference between soluble (i.e., oats, nuts, beans), which forms a gel as it moves through your system, and insoluble fiber (i.e., green leafy vegetables, seeds, bran), which moves through untouched from its original form. Both are important for your health.
- Vegetables should comprise a very large portion of your diet. They are not a side dish. To keep protein high, incorporate beans and tofu into your meatless meals.
- Take a multivitamin daily to make sure you're not depriving yourself of nutrients.
- You may want to add extra Vitamin D (1000 mg) and fish oil to protect yourself from disease and help you lose weight.

- Don't be afraid to special order at any restaurant or catering hall. Instruct waitstaff on what you want: grilled chicken salad, an egg white omelet, etc.
- Have your waiter bring a takeaway carton along with your entrée. Cut your meal in half (at least) immediately and put the second half in the carton so you're not tempted. Enjoy it later!
- Do NOT eat until you're full. Eat only until you're not hungry anymore. Eat to satisfaction—not overindulgence or discomfort.
- Reached a goal? Reward yourself—but not with food. Buy something small that you've wanted. Go walking with friends. Take a day off. Get a new gadget. Get a pedicure. Pamper yourself!
- Snack on fruits and vegetables (grape tomatoes, celery, carrots), as well as proteins like hard-boiled eggs, tuna, hummus, fat-free Greek yogurt.
- Remove skin from poultry before eating.
- Use Canadian bacon instead of regular bacon.
- Replace mayo and sour cream with fat-free yogurt.
- Eat fruit instead of drinking fruit juice. You'll get more fiber and less sugar.
- Clean out the fridge and the cupboards. Replace tempting items with healthful alternatives.

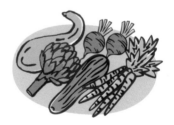

portion control

As mentioned earlier, food industry portions are out of control. Many people would be surprised to see a proper portion size compared to what is served in the average restaurant.

Here are some guidelines that may help you visualize proper portion sizes:

Protein/meat	3 oz/85g (size of your palm or a deck of cards)
Carbs/pasta/rice/potato	1/2 cup/approx. 50-100g (size of a tennis ball cut in half)
Fruits	1 cup/approx. 150g (size of a tennis ball)
Cheese	1 oz/28g (size of 4 dice or your thumb)
Bagel	Average serving: hockey puck size
Potato	Medium serving: size of a computer mouse
Peanut butter/butter	1 tsp/approx. 23g (the tip of your thumb)
Bread	1 slice
Pancake	1 (size of a CD/DVD)
Vegetables	1/2 cup cooked/approx. 75g (size of a tennis ball cut in half)
Lettuce	1 cup/47g (4 leaves)
Milk/yogurt	1 cup/240mL (size of a tennis ball)
Nuts	8 (handful)

If you're having a hard time judging sizes, consider investing in a food scale. That way you can weigh and portion out food in advance. Do it when you get home from the grocery store. Try putting meats, veggies, and especially snacks in individual storage bags.

nutrition label tips

Nutrition labels contain a wealth of information. Here are things to note:

- Watch the serving size!
- 5% is low and 20% is high for all nutrients.
- 40 calories is low, 100 is moderate, and 400 is high.
- Keep saturated fats, sodium, and sugar LOW.
- Keep protein and fiber HIGH.
- Keep in mind Nutrition Facts are based on a 2,000 calorie/day diet—adjust accordingly.

basal metabolic rate

Welcome to your Basal Metabolic Rate! Your BMR indicates the calories your body needs per day to survive without moving. If you're awake and sitting, but not exercising, multiply that number by 1.2—the result is the amount of calories you need to maintain weight. To lose weight, you'll need to cut calories and increase exercise in order to maintain muscle mass. If you don't ingest enough calories for the day, you'll do more harm than good. In general, if you're trying to lose weight, aim for a loss of 1 to 2 pounds a week, no more.

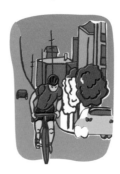

Here's the formula:

> **Women: BMR = 655 + (4.35 x weight in pounds) +
> (4.7 x height in inches) - (4.7 x age in years)**
> **or metric:** 655.1 + (9.56 x weight in kg) +
> (1.85 x height in cm) - (4.68 x age in years)
>
> **Men: BMR = 66 + (6.23 x weight in pounds) +
> (12.7 x height in inches) - (6.8 x age in years)**
> **or metric:** 66.5 + (13.75 x weight in kg) +
> (5 x height in cm) - (6.76 x age in years)

daily recommended caloric intake

Estimate the amount of calories you need to maintain your current weight with the calculator at www.bodybuilding.com/fun/macronutcal. htm.

If you reduce net calories (by eating 500 fewer calories a day and/or exercising), you'll be able to lose 1 pound a week. You need 3,500 fewer calories than required by your BMR to burn off a pound (500 x 7 days = 3,500 calories).

> **Note:** Consuming too few calories will not necessarily get you to your goal faster. If you're not eating enough, your body will lower your BMR in order to conserve its fat stores, so instead of needing the 1,500 calories a day, you may only require 1,000 calories. So if you're consuming 1,200, that may be 200 too many, and you may actually gain weight! See what a tricky business this can be? At that level, your body will also be cannibalizing its own muscle mass to feed itself. So you won't necessarily lose fat, but quite probably muscle. And the more muscle lost, the lower your metabolic rate, and the fewer calories you need, compounding the vicious cycle.

THE SKINNY ON FITNESS
body mass index

The dreaded Body Mass Index! A good indicator of body fatness, your BMI should stay below 25. The formulas below tell how to find yours. Height is measured without shoes and weight without clothes.

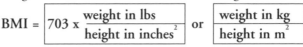

$$\text{BMI} = \boxed{703 \text{ x } \frac{\text{weight in lbs}}{\text{height in inches}^2}} \text{ or } \boxed{\frac{\text{weight in kg}}{\text{height in m}^2}}$$

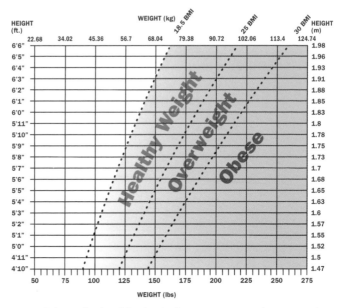

Here are guidelines for healthy body fat percentages, by age and gender. You can ascertain your body fat with a specialized scale or with help from a personal trainer.*

AGE	WOMEN	MEN
20–39	21% to 32%	8% to 19%
40–59	23% to 33%	11% to 21%
60 and up	24% to 35%	13% to 24%

*In addition, BMI should be between 18.5 and 24.9

heart smart exercise
resting heart rate (RHR) vs. maximum heart rate

In order to determine your RHR, first take your pulse, best done when you get up in the morning. Simply place your forefinger and middle finger on your wrist pulse point. Count the number of pulses in a given time period (i.e., count for 10 seconds, and multiply that number by 6 to get your beats per minute. Or count for 30 seconds and multiply by 2). That's your RHR. It should be between 50 and 100. Most people have an RHR around 70. The lower your RHR, the better your cardio-vascular health. The more active you are, the lower your RHR will get.

You want to get your heart rate up during activity to burn more calories. Men, your Maximum Heart Rate is 220 minus your age. If you're 33, that would be 187 beats per minute (220 – 33 = 187 MHR). Women, the latest information says that your MHR should be 206 minus 88% of your age. Meaning, if you're 33, that would be 177 beats per minute (206 – (33 x .88) = 177 MHR). For optimum fat-burning benefits during exercise, keep that heart rate between 65% and 85% of your MHR. Do the math, multiplying your MHR by .65 or .85, to figure out where your heart rate should be for the best fat burn.

The faster your heart beats, the speedier your metabolism. (That's why most "diet" pills have caffeine in them.)

Now, while the "fat-burning zone" will burn a higher percentage of fat, the cardio zone will burn more calories and a higher *amount* of fat. Thus, if you can keep it up in the cardio zone, you'll see better results.

burning calories

Moderate Physical Activity	Approximate Calories/Hr*
Hiking	370
Light gardening/yard work	330
Dancing	330
Golf (walking and carrying clubs)	330
Bicycling (<10 mph or 16 kph)	290
Walking (3.5 mph or 5.6 kph)	280
Weight lifting (general light workout)	220
Stretching	180
Vigorous Physical Activity	**Approximate Calories/Hr***
Running/jogging (5 mph or 8 kph)	590
Bicycling (>10 mph or 16 kph)	590
Swimming (slow freestyle laps)	510
Aerobics	480
Walking (4.5 mph or 7.2 kph)	460
Heavy yard work (chopping wood)	440
Weight lifting (vigorous effort)	440
Basketball (vigorous)	440

*Calories burned per hour are based on a 154-pound person. Calories burned will be higher for those who weigh more than 154 pounds (70 kg) and lower for those who weigh less.

cardio: what have you done for me lately?

What's the big deal about cardio? Put simply, this is what burns calories. Ate that chocolate cake and want to burn off the extra 500 calories? Do some quick sprints on the treadmill for 30–45 minutes. Or do some interval training on the elliptical machine. Cardio activity speeds up your heart rate, increases oxygen intake, and revs your metabolism. You can do a cardio workout at the gym or outside.

levels & duration

While you can set the difficulty "level" you're working at in the gym, how can you judge the level outside? Simple—just pay attention to how you breathe and if you sweat.

Level	Calories burned per minute	Breathing	Sweating
Easy	3–5	Breathing normal, can sing and carry on conversation	No
Moderate	6–8	Breathing deep, can't sing, but can talk in bursts	After 10 minutes
Difficult	9–12	Breathing frequent and deep, can't sing, difficult to talk	After 3–5 minutes

When you first begin exercising, you may drop a nice chunk of weight almost immediately. I like to think of this as a gift. Yes, it's mostly water weight, but it sure is encouraging! Just don't give up if you don't see the same results in the second and third week. By that time, you're actually burning fat stores—that takes longer to lose than water.

You should be doing 30–60 minutes of cardio activity a day, each day, if you're trying to lose weight. If you're trying to maintain, you can drop that down to 3–4 times a week.

weight training: pump yourself up!

OK, if cardio is what burns the calories, why bother with weight training? Because weight training is what keeps off the fat and builds muscle. The more muscle mass you have, the higher your BMR, and the more calories you'll burn—*even when you're not exercising.* Ah, this sounds like something you want to do, right? Right!

Ladies, do not be afraid of free weights. You will not look like the Terminator because you lift a 10-pound (4.5 kg) dumbbell a few times a week. You do not have the testosterone to bulk up like that. You'll just get sleek, attractive muscle definition. Nice!

Aim to work different groups of muscles every other day, allowing a day of rest between each session for a particular group. For example: Work the legs on Day 1, but not again until Day 3.

sets & reps

Perform each set 3 times, for 8–15 repetitions. Build up to it. Make sure the weight is such that you are straining to do the last few, otherwise, it's not heavy enough. Rest for 30–60 seconds after each set.

You might experiment with super sets. Instead of resting between sets, simply reduce the weight and continue doing reps until 3 sets are complete. Then rest.

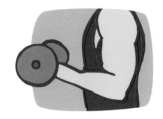

fitness tips & tricks

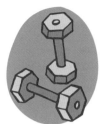

- Exercise twice a day—once in the morning or around noon, and again in the late afternoon or evening. It needn't be for long periods.

- Exercising in the morning will jump-start your metabolism for the day.

- Use interval training: After warming up, ramp up to do 1 minute at your highest level, 2 at medium level, then go back to 1 at high, 2 at medium, etc., throughout the workout. The speed interval will raise your heart rate and trick your body into burning at a rate almost as high as doing the hardest level the entire time.

- Even if the scale doesn't change, it doesn't mean you're not successful. You may have lost inches, fat, and/or improved your health! Fabulous!

- Get enough sleep—at least 7 to 7.5 hours a night.

And for your own sake, do not give up. Be just as stubborn, if not more so, as the fat you're trying to lose.

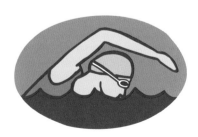

HELPFUL ONLINE RESOURCES
nutrition information:
www.usda.gov
www.health.gov/dietaryguidelines
www.caloriecontrol.org
www.choosemyplate.gov
www.webmd.com
nutritiondata.self.com
www.glycemicindex.com
www.cspinet.org
www.hsph.harvard.edu/nutritionsource
www.myfooddiary.com
www.livestrong.com/myplate
www.food.gov.uk
www.nutrition.org.uk
www.gov.uk/government/policies/obesity-and-healthy-eating

fitness:
www.mensfitness.com
www.fitnessmagazine.com
www.nhs.uk/livewell/fitness
www.muscleandfitness.com
www.acsm.org
www.acefitness.org
www.nasm.org
www.prohealth.com

support:
www.niddk.nih.gov/health-information/weight-management/
health-tips-adults
www.weightwatchers.com
www.jennycraig.com
www.ediets.com
www.hungry-girl.com

DAILY
&WEEKLY
food
&fitness
LOG PAGES

*To be successful, you must dedicate
yourself 100% to your training,
diet, and mental approach.*

ARNOLD SCHWARZENEGGER

FOOD LOG

Day	Date	Week #

	Portion	Calories (kcal)	Fat (g)	Saturated Fat (g)	Sodium (mg)	Carbs (g)	Fiber (g)	Protein (g)	Other
BREAKFAST Time:									
Breakfast Totals →									
SNACK Time:									
Snack Totals →									
LUNCH Time:									
Lunch Totals →									
SNACK Time:									
Snack Totals →									
DINNER Time:									
Dinner Totals →									
SNACK Time:									
Snack Totals →									
Daily Totals →									

DAILY FOOD GOALS

target	actual	
		calories
		protein (g)
		carbs (g)
		fat (g)

water (8 oz glasses)

☐ ☐ ☐ ☐ ☐ ☐ ☐ ☐

fruits + vegetables (servings)

☐ ☐ ☐ ☐ ☐ ☐ ☐ ☐ ☐ ☐

FITNESS LOG

CARDIO/OTHER	Time of Day	Heart Rate	Duration	Speed	Level	Intensity	Other	Calories (kcal) Used
Calorie Totals								

WEIGHTS	Time of Day	Muscle Group	Reps	Sets	Duration	Intensity	Other	Calories (kcal) Used
Calorie Totals								
Total Calories Burned								

Calories Consumed	–	Calories Used	=	Net Calories	–	BMR (Basal Metabolic Rate)	=	Net Calorie Deficit

Vitamins/Supplements	Dosage	Quantity

mood

☹ 2 3 4 5 6 7 ☺

energy level

1 2 3 4 5 6 7 8

A 3,500 calorie deficit will equal 1 lb of weight loss.

Notes/Journal

FOOD LOG

Day	Date	Week #

	Portion	Calories (kcal)	Fat (g)	Saturated Fat (g)	Sodium (mg)	Carbs (g)	Fiber (g)	Protein (g)	Other
BREAKFAST Time:									
Breakfast Totals →									
SNACK Time:									
Snack Totals →									
LUNCH Time:									
Lunch Totals →									
SNACK Time:									
Snack Totals →									
DINNER Time:									
Dinner Totals →									
SNACK Time:									
Snack Totals →									
Daily Totals →									

DAILY FOOD GOALS

target	actual	
		calories
		protein (g)
		carbs (g)
		fat (g)

water (8 oz glasses)

☐ ☐ ☐ ☐ ☐ ☐ ☐ ☐

fruits + vegetables (servings)

☐ ☐ ☐ ☐ ☐ ☐ ☐ ☐ ☐ ☐

FITNESS LOG

CARDIO/OTHER	Time of Day	Heart Rate	Duration	Speed	Level	Intensity	Other	Calories (kcal) Used
Calorie Totals								

WEIGHTS	Time of Day	Muscle Group	Reps	Sets	Duration	Intensity	Other	Calories (kcal) Used
Calorie Totals								
Total Calories Burned								

Calories Consumed	-	Calories Used	=	Net Calories	-	BMR (Basal Metabolic Rate)	=	Net Calorie Deficit

Vitamins/Supplements	Dosage	Quantity

mood

☹ 2 3 4 5 6 7 ☺

energy level

1 2 3 4 5 6 7 8

A 3,500 calorie deficit will equal 1 lb of weight loss.

Notes/Journal

FOOD LOG

	Day	Date	Week #

			Calories (kcal)	Fat (g)	Saturated Fat (g)	Sodium (mg)	Carbs (g)	Fiber (g)	Protein (g)	Othe
BREAKFAST Time:		Portion								
Breakfast Totals	→									
SNACK Time:										
Snack Totals	→									
LUNCH Time:										
Lunch Totals	→									
SNACK Time:										
Snack Totals	→									
DINNER Time:										
Dinner Totals	→									
SNACK Time:										
Snack Totals	→									
Daily Totals	→									

DAILY FOOD GOALS

target	actual	
		calories
		protein (g)
		carbs (g)
		fat (g)

water (8 oz glasses)

☐☐☐☐☐☐☐☐

fruits + vegetables (servings)

☐☐☐☐☐☐☐☐☐

FITNESS LOG

CARDIO/OTHER	Time of Day	Heart Rate	Duration	Speed	Level	Intensity	Other	Calories (kcal) Used
Calorie Totals								

WEIGHTS	Time of Day	Muscle Group	Reps	Sets	Duration	Intensity	Other	Calories (kcal) Used
Calorie Totals								

Total Calories Burned

Calories Consumed	−	Calories Used	=	Net Calories	−	BMR (Basal Metabolic Rate)	=	Net Calorie Deficit

Vitamins/Supplements	Dosage	Quantity	mood	A 3,500
			☹ 2 3 4 5 6 7 ☺	calorie deficit will equal
			energy level	1 lb of
			1 2 3 4 5 6 7 8	weight loss.

Notes/Journal

FOOD LOG

Day	Date	Week #

	Portion	Calories (kcal)	Fat (g)	Saturated Fat (g)	Sodium (mg)	Carbs (g)	Fiber (g)	Protein (g)	Other
BREAKFAST Time:									
Breakfast Totals →									
SNACK Time:									
Snack Totals →									
LUNCH Time:									
Lunch Totals →									
SNACK Time:									
Snack Totals →									
DINNER Time:									
Dinner Totals →									
SNACK Time:									
Snack Totals →									
Daily Totals →									

DAILY FOOD GOALS

target	actual	
		calories
		protein (g)
		carbs (g)
		fat (g)

water (8 oz glasses)
☐☐☐☐☐☐☐☐

fruits + vegetables (servings)
☐☐☐☐☐☐☐☐☐☐

FITNESS LOG

CARDIO/OTHER	Time of Day	Heart Rate	Duration	Speed	Level	Intensity	Other	Calories (kcal) Used
Calorie Totals								

WEIGHTS	Time of Day	Muscle Group	Reps	Sets	Duration	Intensity	Other	Calories (kcal) Used
Calorie Totals								

Total Calories Burned

Calories Consumed	-	Calories Used	=	Net Calories	-	BMR (Basal Metabolic Rate)	=	Net Calorie Deficit

Vitamins/Supplements	Dosage	Quantity

mood

☹ 2 3 4 5 6 7 ☺

energy level

1 2 3 4 5 6 7 8

A 3,500 calorie deficit will equal 1 lb of weight loss.

Notes/Journal

FOOD LOG

Day	Date	Week #

	Calories (kcal)	Fat (g)	Saturated Fat (g)	Sodium (mg)	Carbs (g)	Fiber (g)	Protein (g)	Other
BREAKFAST Time: Portion								
Breakfast Totals →								
SNACK Time:								
Snack Totals →								
LUNCH Time:								
Lunch Totals →								
SNACK Time:								
Snack Totals →								
DINNER Time:								
Dinner Totals →								
SNACK Time:								
Snack Totals →								
Daily Totals →								

DAILY FOOD GOALS

	target	actual
calories		
protein (g)		
carbs (g)		
fat (g)		

water (8 oz glasses)

☐ ☐ ☐ ☐ ☐ ☐ ☐ ☐

fruits + vegetables (servings)

☐ ☐ ☐ ☐ ☐ ☐ ☐ ☐ ☐

FITNESS LOG

CARDIO/OTHER	Time of Day	Heart Rate	Duration	Speed	Level	Intensity	Other	Calories (kcal) Used
Calorie Totals								

WEIGHTS	Time of Day	Muscle Group	Reps	Sets	Duration	Intensity	Other	Calories (kcal) Used
Calorie Totals								

Total Calories Burned

Calories Consumed	−	Calories Used	=	Net Calories	−	BMR (Basal Metabolic Rate)	=	Net Calorie Deficit

Vitamins/Supplements	Dosage	Quantity

mood

☹ 2 3 4 5 6 7 ☺

energy level

1 2 3 4 5 6 7 8

A 3,500 calorie deficit will equal 1 lb of weight loss.

Notes/Journal

FOOD LOG

Day		Date		Week #

			Calories (kcal)	Fat (g)	Saturated Fat (g)	Sodium (mg)	Carbs (g)	Fiber (g)	Protein (g)	Other
BREAKFAST Time:		Portion								
Breakfast Totals →										
SNACK Time:										
Snack Totals →										
LUNCH Time:										
Lunch Totals →										
SNACK Time:										
Snack Totals →										
DINNER Time:										
Dinner Totals →										
SNACK Time:										
Snack Totals →										
Daily Totals →										

DAILY FOOD GOALS

	target	actual
calories		
protein (g)		
carbs (g)		
fat (g)		

water (8 oz glasses)

☐ ☐ ☐ ☐ ☐ ☐ ☐ ☐

fruits + vegetables (servings)

☐ ☐ ☐ ☐ ☐ ☐ ☐ ☐ ☐

FITNESS LOG

CARDIO/OTHER	Time of Day	Heart Rate	Duration	Speed	Level	Intensity	Other	Calories (kcal) Used
Calorie Totals								

WEIGHTS	Time of Day	Muscle Group	Reps	Sets	Duration	Intensity	Other	Calories (kcal) Used
Calorie Totals								

Total Calories Burned

Calories Consumed		Calories Used		Net Calories		BMR (Basal Metabolic Rate)		Net Calorie Deficit
	-		=		-		=	

Vitamins/Supplements	Dosage	Quantity	
			mood
			☹ 2 3 4 5 6 7 ☺
			energy level
			1 2 3 4 5 6 7 8

A 3,500 calorie deficit will equal 1 lb of weight loss.

Notes/Journal

FOOD LOG

Day	Date	Week #

	Calories (kcal)	Fat (g)	Saturated Fat (g)	Sodium (mg)	Carbs (g)	Fiber (g)	Protein (g)	Other
BREAKFAST Time: Portion								
Breakfast Totals →								
SNACK Time:								
Snack Totals →								
LUNCH Time:								
Lunch Totals →								
SNACK Time:								
Snack Totals →								
DINNER Time:								
Dinner Totals →								
SNACK Time:								
Snack Totals →								
Daily Totals →								

DAILY FOOD GOALS

target	actual	
		calories
		protein (g)
		carbs (g)
		fat (g)

water (8 oz glasses)

☐ ☐ ☐ ☐ ☐ ☐ ☐ ☐

fruits + vegetables (servings)

☐ ☐ ☐ ☐ ☐ ☐ ☐ ☐ ☐

FITNESS LOG

CARDIO/OTHER	Time of Day	Heart Rate	Duration	Speed	Level	Intensity	Other	Calories (kcal) Used
Calorie Totals								

WEIGHTS	Time of Day	Muscle Group	Reps	Sets	Duration	Intensity	Other	Calories (kcal) Used
Calorie Totals								

Total Calories Burned

Calories Consumed	−	Calories Used	=	Net Calories	−	BMR (Basal Metabolic Rate)	=	Net Calorie Deficit

Vitamins/Supplements	Dosage	Quantity	mood	
			☹ 2 3 4 5 6 7 ☺	A 3,500 calorie deficit
			energy level	will equal 1 lb of
			1 2 3 4 5 6 7 8	weight loss.

Notes/Journal

WEEKLY PROGRESS

STATS

	Weight	BMI	BMR	Heart Rate	Cholesterol	Blood Sugar	Other
Last Week							
Current							

MEASUREMENTS

	Neck	Shoulder	Chest	Waist	Hip	Thigh	Calf	Arm	Other
Last Week									
Current									

Notes/Journal

GOALS FOR NEXT WEEK

DAILY CALORIE DEFICIT

Day 1		Day 5	
Day 2		Day 6	
Day 3		Day 7	
Day 4		Weekly Total	

Waist Hip Ratio

Women <.7
Men   <.9

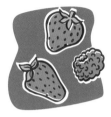

You can learn to listen to your inner self,
get to know what's good for you
and love the body you have.

SALMA HAYEK

TIP OF THE WEEK

The real issue is not losing weight—people can cut back on calories and lose weight on almost any diet—but keeping weight off over the long run. Thus, it is more important to find a way of eating that you can stay with for the rest of your life.

—Dr. Walter Willett,
Harvard School of Public Health

FOOD LOG

	Day		Date		Week #	

		Calories (kcal)	Fat (g)	Saturated Fat (g)	Sodium (mg)	Carbs (g)	Fiber (g)	Protein (g)	Other
BREAKFAST Time:	Portion								
Breakfast Totals →									
SNACK Time:									
Snack Totals →									
LUNCH Time:									
Lunch Totals →									
SNACK Time:									
Snack Totals →									
DINNER Time:									
Dinner Totals →									
SNACK Time:									
Snack Totals →									
Daily Totals →									

DAILY FOOD GOALS

	target	actual	
			calories
			protein (g)
			carbs (g)
			fat (g)

water (8 oz glasses)

☐ ☐ ☐ ☐ ☐ ☐ ☐ ☐

fruits + vegetables (servings)

☐ ☐ ☐ ☐ ☐ ☐ ☐ ☐ ☐ ☐

FITNESS LOG

CARDIO/OTHER	Time of Day	Heart Rate	Duration	Speed	Level	Intensity	Other	Calories (kcal) Used
Calorie Totals								

WEIGHTS	Time of Day	Muscle Group	Reps	Sets	Duration	Intensity	Other	Calories (kcal) Used
Calorie Totals								

Total Calories Burned

Calories Consumed		Calories Used		Net Calories		BMR (Basal Metabolic Rate)		Net Calorie Deficit
	−		=		−		=	

Vitamins/Supplements	Dosage	Quantity

mood

☹ 2 3 4 5 6 7 ☺

energy level

1 2 3 4 5 6 7 8

A 3,500 calorie deficit will equal 1 lb of weight loss.

Notes/Journal

FOOD LOG

Day	Date	Week #

	Portion	Calories (kcal)	Fat (g)	Saturated Fat (g)	Sodium (mg)	Carbs (g)	Fiber (g)	Protein (g)	Other
BREAKFAST Time:									
Breakfast Totals →									
SNACK Time:									
Snack Totals →									
LUNCH Time:									
Lunch Totals →									
SNACK Time:									
Snack Totals →									
DINNER Time:									
Dinner Totals →									
SNACK Time:									
Snack Totals →									
Daily Totals →									

DAILY FOOD GOALS

target	actual	
		calories
		protein (g)
		carbs (g)
		fat (g)

water (8 oz glasses)

☐ ☐ ☐ ☐ ☐ ☐ ☐ ☐

fruits + vegetables (servings)

☐ ☐ ☐ ☐ ☐ ☐ ☐ ☐ ☐

FITNESS LOG

CARDIO/OTHER	Time of Day	Heart Rate	Duration	Speed	Level	Intensity	Other	Calories (kcal) Used
Calorie Totals								

WEIGHTS	Time of Day	Muscle Group	Reps	Sets	Duration	Intensity	Other	Calories (kcal) Used
Calorie Totals								

Total Calories Burned

Calories Consumed	−	Calories Used	=	Net Calories	−	BMR (Basal Metabolic Rate)	=	Net Calorie Deficit

Vitamins/Supplements	Dosage	Quantity

mood
☹ 2 3 4 5 6 7 ☺

energy level
1 2 3 4 5 6 7 8

A 3,500 calorie deficit will equal 1 lb of weight loss.

Notes/Journal

FOOD LOG

Day	Date	Week #

			Calories (kcal)	Fat (g)	Saturated Fat (g)	Sodium (mg)	Carbs (g)	Fiber (g)	Protein (g)	Other
BREAKFAST	Time:	Portion								
Breakfast Totals	→									
SNACK	Time:									
Snack Totals	→									
LUNCH	Time:									
Lunch Totals	→									
SNACK	Time:									
Snack Totals	→									
DINNER	Time:									
Dinner Totals	→									
SNACK	Time:									
Snack Totals	→									
Daily Totals	→									

DAILY FOOD GOALS

target	actual	
		calories
		protein (g)
		carbs (g)
		fat (g)

water (8 oz glasses)

☐☐☐☐☐☐☐☐

fruits + vegetables (servings)

☐☐☐☐☐☐☐☐☐☐

FITNESS LOG

CARDIO/OTHER	Time of Day	Heart Rate	Duration	Speed	Level	Intensity	Other	Calories (kcal) Used
Calorie Totals								

WEIGHTS	Time of Day	Muscle Group	Reps	Sets	Duration	Intensity	Other	Calories (kcal) Used
Calorie Totals								

Total Calories Burned

Calories Consumed		Calories Used		Net Calories		BMR (Basal Metabolic Rate)		Net Calorie Deficit
	−		=		−		=	

Vitamins/Supplements	Dosage	Quantity

mood

☹ 2 3 4 5 6 7 ☺

energy level

1 2 3 4 5 6 7 8

A 3,500 calorie deficit will equal 1 lb of weight loss.

Notes/Journal

FOOD LOG

	Day		Date		Week #	

			Calories (kcal)	Fat (g)	Saturated Fat (g)	Sodium (mg)	Carbs (g)	Fiber (g)	Protein (g)	Othe
BREAKFAST Time:		Portion								
Breakfast Totals →										
SNACK Time:										
Snack Totals →										
LUNCH Time:										
Lunch Totals →										
SNACK Time:										
Snack Totals →										
DINNER Time:										
Dinner Totals →										
SNACK Time:										
Snack Totals →										
Daily Totals →										

DAILY FOOD GOALS

target	actual	
		calories
		protein (g)
		carbs (g)
		fat (g)

water (8 oz glasses)

☐ ☐ ☐ ☐ ☐ ☐ ☐ ☐

fruits + vegetables (servings)

☐ ☐ ☐ ☐ ☐ ☐ ☐ ☐ ☐ ☐

FITNESS LOG

CARDIO/OTHER	Time of Day	Heart Rate	Duration	Speed	Level	Intensity	Other	Calories (kcal) Used
Calorie Totals								

WEIGHTS	Time of Day	Muscle Group	Reps	Sets	Duration	Intensity	Other	Calories (kcal) Used
Calorie Totals								
Total Calories Burned								

Calories Consumed	−	Calories Used	=	Net Calories	−	BMR (Basal Metabolic Rate)	=	Net Calorie Deficit

Vitamins/Supplements	Dosage	Quantity

mood

☹ 2 3 4 5 6 7 ☺

energy level

1 2 3 4 5 6 7 8

A 3,500 calorie deficit will equal 1 lb of weight loss.

Notes/Journal

FOOD LOG

| | Day | | Date | | Week # |

	Portion	Calories (kcal)	Fat (g)	Saturated Fat (g)	Sodium (mg)	Carbs (g)	Fiber (g)	Protein (g)	Other
BREAKFAST Time:	Portion								
Breakfast Totals →									
SNACK Time:									
Snack Totals →									
LUNCH Time:									
Lunch Totals →									
SNACK Time:									
Snack Totals →									
DINNER Time:									
Dinner Totals →									
SNACK Time:									
Snack Totals →									
Daily Totals →									

DAILY FOOD GOALS

target	actual	
		calories
		protein (g)
		carbs (g)
		fat (g)

water (8 oz glasses)

☐ ☐ ☐ ☐ ☐ ☐ ☐ ☐

fruits + vegetables (servings)

☐ ☐ ☐ ☐ ☐ ☐ ☐ ☐ ☐

FITNESS LOG

CARDIO/OTHER	Time of Day	Heart Rate	Duration	Speed	Level	Intensity	Other	Calories (kcal) Used
Calorie Totals								

WEIGHTS	Time of Day	Muscle Group	Reps	Sets	Duration	Intensity	Other	Calories (kcal) Used
Calorie Totals								
Total Calories Burned								

Calories Consumed	–	Calories Used	=	Net Calories	–	BMR (Basal Metabolic Rate)	=	Net Calorie Deficit

Vitamins/Supplements	Dosage	Quantity

mood

☹ 2 3 4 5 6 7 ☺

energy level

1 2 3 4 5 6 7 8

A 3,500 calorie deficit will equal 1 lb of weight loss.

Notes/Journal

FOOD LOG

| Day | Date | Week # |

		Portion	Calories (kcal)	Fat (g)	Saturated Fat (g)	Sodium (mg)	Carbs (g)	Fiber (g)	Protein (g)	Other
BREAKFAST Time:		Portion								
Breakfast Totals →										
SNACK Time:										
Snack Totals →										
LUNCH Time:										
Lunch Totals →										
SNACK Time:										
Snack Totals →										
DINNER Time:										
Dinner Totals →										
SNACK Time:										
Snack Totals →										
Daily Totals →										

DAILY FOOD GOALS

	target	actual
calories		
protein (g)		
carbs (g)		
fat (g)		

water (8 oz glasses)

☐ ☐ ☐ ☐ ☐ ☐ ☐ ☐

fruits + vegetables (servings)

☐ ☐ ☐ ☐ ☐ ☐ ☐ ☐ ☐

FITNESS LOG

CARDIO/OTHER	Time of Day	Heart Rate	Duration	Speed	Level	Intensity	Other	Calories (kcal) Used
Calorie Totals								

WEIGHTS	Time of Day	Muscle Group	Reps	Sets	Duration	Intensity	Other	Calories (kcal) Used
Calorie Totals								
Total Calories Burned								

Calories Consumed − Calories Used = Net Calories − BMR (Basal Metabolic Rate) = Net Calorie Deficit

Vitamins/Supplements	Dosage	Quantity

mood
☹ 2 3 4 5 6 7 ☺
energy level
1 2 3 4 5 6 7 8

A 3,500 calorie deficit will equal 1 lb of weight loss.

Notes/Journal

FOOD LOG

| Day | | Date | | Week # |

	Calories (kcal)	Fat (g)	Saturated Fat (g)	Sodium (mg)	Carbs (g)	Fiber (g)	Protein (g)	Other
BREAKFAST Time: Portion								
Breakfast Totals →								
SNACK Time:								
Snack Totals →								
LUNCH Time:								
Lunch Totals →								
SNACK Time:								
Snack Totals →								
DINNER Time:								
Dinner Totals →								
SNACK Time:								
Snack Totals →								
Daily Totals →								

DAILY FOOD GOALS

target	actual	
		calories
		protein (g)
		carbs (g)
		fat (g)

water (8 oz glasses)

☐ ☐ ☐ ☐ ☐ ☐ ☐ ☐

fruits + vegetables (servings)

☐ ☐ ☐ ☐ ☐ ☐ ☐ ☐ ☐

FITNESS LOG

CARDIO/OTHER	Time of Day	Heart Rate	Duration	Speed	Level	Intensity	Other	Calories (kcal) Used
Calorie Totals								

WEIGHTS	Time of Day	Muscle Group	Reps	Sets	Duration	Intensity	Other	Calories (kcal) Used
Calorie Totals								
Total Calories Burned								

Calories Consumed	–	Calories Used	=	Net Calories	–	BMR (Basal Metabolic Rate)	=	Net Calorie Deficit

Vitamins/Supplements	Dosage	Quantity

mood

☹ 2 3 4 5 6 7 ☺

energy level

1 2 3 4 5 6 7 8

A 3,500 calorie deficit will equal 1 lb of weight loss.

Notes/Journal

WEEKLY PROGRESS

	Weight	BMI	BMR	Heart Rate	Cholesterol	Blood Sugar	Other
STATS							
Last Week							
Current							

	Neck	Shoulder	Chest	Waist	Hip	Thigh	Calf	Arm	Other
MEASUREMENTS									
Last Week									
Current									

Notes/Journal

GOALS FOR NEXT WEEK

DAILY CALORIE DEFICIT

Day 1		Day 5	
Day 2		Day 6	
Day 3		Day 7	
Day 4		Weekly Total	

Waist Hip Ratio

Women <.7
Men   <.9

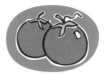

*With every wish that you make comes the power
to make it come true. But it is up to you to
provide the work that will make it a reality.
Are you using your power to make
your wishes come true today?*

LIBBY ROSENAU

TIP OF THE WEEK

Research published in the last two years shows
that certain slow activities—like gentle yoga or
gardening—can reduce your stress level and blood
pressure and improve your body's ability to regulate sugar.

—Chrystle Fiedler

FOOD LOG

Day	Date	Week #

	Portion	Calories (kcal)	Fat (g)	Saturated Fat (g)	Sodium (mg)	Carbs (g)	Fiber (g)	Protein (g)	Other
BREAKFAST Time:									
Breakfast Totals →									
SNACK Time:									
Snack Totals →									
LUNCH Time:									
Lunch Totals →									
SNACK Time:									
Snack Totals →									
DINNER Time:									
Dinner Totals →									
SNACK Time:									
Snack Totals →									
Daily Totals →									

DAILY FOOD GOALS

	target	actual
calories		
protein (g)		
carbs (g)		
fat (g)		

water (8 oz glasses)

☐ ☐ ☐ ☐ ☐ ☐ ☐ ☐

fruits + vegetables (servings)

☐ ☐ ☐ ☐ ☐ ☐ ☐ ☐ ☐ ☐

FITNESS LOG

CARDIO/OTHER	Time of Day	Heart Rate	Duration	Speed	Level	Intensity	Other	Calories (kcal) Used
Calorie Totals								

WEIGHTS	Time of Day	Muscle Group	Reps	Sets	Duration	Intensity	Other	Calories (kcal) Used
Calorie Totals								

Total Calories Burned

Calories Consumed		Calories Used		Net Calories		BMR (Basal Metabolic Rate)		Net Calorie Deficit
	−		=		−		=	

Vitamins/Supplements	Dosage	Quantity

mood

☹ 2 3 4 5 6 7 ☺

energy level

1 2 3 4 5 6 7 8

A 3,500 calorie deficit will equal 1 lb of weight loss.

Notes/Journal

FOOD LOG

		Day		Date		Week #	

	Portion	Calories (kcal)	Fat (g)	Saturated Fat (g)	Sodium (mg)	Carbs (g)	Fiber (g)	Protein (g)	Other
BREAKFAST Time:									
Breakfast Totals →									
SNACK Time:									
Snack Totals →									
LUNCH Time:									
Lunch Totals →									
SNACK Time:									
Snack Totals →									
DINNER Time:									
Dinner Totals →									
SNACK Time:									
Snack Totals →									
Daily Totals →									

DAILY FOOD GOALS

target	actual	
		calories
		protein (g)
		carbs (g)
		fat (g)

water (8 oz glasses)

☐ ☐ ☐ ☐ ☐ ☐ ☐ ☐

fruits + vegetables (servings)

☐ ☐ ☐ ☐ ☐ ☐ ☐ ☐ ☐ ☐

FITNESS LOG

CARDIO/OTHER	Time of Day	Heart Rate	Duration	Speed	Level	Intensity	Other	Calories (kcal) Used
Calorie Totals								

WEIGHTS	Time of Day	Muscle Group	Reps	Sets	Duration	Intensity	Other	Calories (kcal) Used
Calorie Totals								

Total Calories Burned

Calories Consumed	-	Calories Used	=	Net Calories	-	BMR (Basal Metabolic Rate)	=	Net Calorie Deficit

Vitamins/Supplements	Dosage	Quantity

mood

☹ 2 3 4 5 6 7 ☺

energy level

1 2 3 4 5 6 7 8

A 3,500 calorie deficit will equal 1 lb of weight loss.

Notes/Journal

FOOD LOG

Day	Date	Week #

			Calories (kcal)	Fat (g)	Saturated Fat (g)	Sodium (mg)	Carbs (g)	Fiber (g)	Protein (g)	Other
BREAKFAST Time:		Portion								
Breakfast Totals	→									
SNACK Time:										
Snack Totals	→									
LUNCH Time:										
Lunch Totals	→									
SNACK Time:										
Snack Totals	→									
DINNER Time:										
Dinner Totals	→									
SNACK Time:										
Snack Totals	→									
Daily Totals	→									

DAILY FOOD GOALS

target	actual	
		calories
		protein (g)
		carbs (g)
		fat (g)

water (8 oz glasses)

☐ ☐ ☐ ☐ ☐ ☐ ☐ ☐

fruits + vegetables (servings)

☐ ☐ ☐ ☐ ☐ ☐ ☐ ☐ ☐

FITNESS LOG

CARDIO/OTHER	Time of Day	Heart Rate	Duration	Speed	Level	Intensity	Other	Calories (kcal) Used
Calorie Totals								

WEIGHTS	Time of Day	Muscle Group	Reps	Sets	Duration	Intensity	Other	Calories (kcal) Used
Calorie Totals								

Total Calories Burned

Calories Consumed	-	Calories Used	=	Net Calories	-	BMR (Basal Metabolic Rate)	=	Net Calorie Deficit

Vitamins/Supplements	Dosage	Quantity

mood

☹ 2 3 4 5 6 7 ☺

energy level

1 2 3 4 5 6 7 8

A 3,500 calorie deficit will equal 1 lb of weight loss.

Notes/Journal

FOOD LOG

Day	Date	Week #

BREAKFAST Time:	Portion	Calories (kcal)	Fat (g)	Saturated Fat (g)	Sodium (mg)	Carbs (g)	Fiber (g)	Protein (g)	Other
Breakfast Totals →									
SNACK Time:									
Snack Totals →									
LUNCH Time:									
Lunch Totals →									
SNACK Time:									
Snack Totals →									
DINNER Time:									
Dinner Totals →									
SNACK Time:									
Snack Totals →									
Daily Totals →									

DAILY FOOD GOALS

	target	actual
calories		
protein (g)		
carbs (g)		
fat (g)		

water (8 oz glasses)

☐ ☐ ☐ ☐ ☐ ☐ ☐ ☐ ☐

fruits + vegetables (servings)

☐ ☐ ☐ ☐ ☐ ☐ ☐ ☐ ☐ ☐ ☐

FITNESS LOG

CARDIO/OTHER	Time of Day	Heart Rate	Duration	Speed	Level	Intensity	Other	Calories (kcal) Used
Calorie Totals								

WEIGHTS	Time of Day	Muscle Group	Reps	Sets	Duration	Intensity	Other	Calories (kcal) Used
Calorie Totals								

Total Calories Burned

Calories Consumed	−	Calories Used	=	Net Calories	−	BMR (Basal Metabolic Rate)	=	Net Calorie Deficit

Vitamins/Supplements	Dosage	Quantity

mood

☹ 2 3 4 5 6 7 ☺

energy level

1 2 3 4 5 6 7 8

A 3,500 calorie deficit will equal 1 lb of weight loss.

Notes/Journal

FOOD LOG

Day		Date		Week #

	Portion	Calories (kcal)	Fat (g)	Saturated Fat (g)	Sodium (mg)	Carbs (g)	Fiber (g)	Protein (g)	Other
BREAKFAST Time:									
Breakfast Totals →									
SNACK Time:									
Snack Totals →									
LUNCH Time:									
Lunch Totals →									
SNACK Time:									
Snack Totals →									
DINNER Time:									
Dinner Totals →									
SNACK Time:									
Snack Totals →									
Daily Totals →									

DAILY FOOD GOALS

	target	actual	
			calories
			protein (g)
			carbs (g)
			fat (g)

water (8 oz glasses)

☐☐☐☐☐☐☐☐☐

fruits + vegetables (servings)

☐☐☐☐☐☐☐☐☐☐

FITNESS LOG

CARDIO/OTHER	Time of Day	Heart Rate	Duration	Speed	Level	Intensity	Other	Calories (kcal) Used
Calorie Totals								

WEIGHTS	Time of Day	Muscle Group	Reps	Sets	Duration	Intensity	Other	Calories (kcal) Used
Calorie Totals								

Total Calories Burned

Calories Consumed	−	Calories Used	=	Net Calories	−	BMR (Basal Metabolic Rate)	=	Net Calorie Deficit

Vitamins/Supplements	Dosage	Quantity

mood

☹ 2 3 4 5 6 7 ☺

energy level

1 2 3 4 5 6 7 8

A 3,500 calorie deficit will equal 1 lb of weight loss.

Notes/Journal

FOOD LOG

Day	Date	Week #

BREAKFAST Time:	Portion	Calories (kcal)	Fat (g)	Saturated Fat (g)	Sodium (mg)	Carbs (g)	Fiber (g)	Protein (g)	Other
Breakfast Totals →									
SNACK Time:									
Snack Totals →									
LUNCH Time:									
Lunch Totals →									
SNACK Time:									
Snack Totals →									
DINNER Time:									
Dinner Totals →									
SNACK Time:									
Snack Totals →									
Daily Totals →									

DAILY FOOD GOALS

	target	actual
calories		
protein (g)		
carbs (g)		
fat (g)		

water (8 oz glasses)

☐ ☐ ☐ ☐ ☐ ☐ ☐ ☐

fruits + vegetables (servings)

☐ ☐ ☐ ☐ ☐ ☐ ☐ ☐ ☐ ☐

FITNESS LOG

CARDIO/OTHER	Time of Day	Heart Rate	Duration	Speed	Level	Intensity	Other	Calories (kcal) Used
Calorie Totals								

WEIGHTS	Time of Day	Muscle Group	Reps	Sets	Duration	Intensity	Other	Calories (kcal) Used
Calorie Totals								
Total Calories Burned								

Calories Consumed	−	Calories Used	=	Net Calories	−	BMR (Basal Metabolic Rate)	=	Net Calorie Deficit

Vitamins/Supplements	Dosage	Quantity

mood

☹ 2 3 4 5 6 7 ☺

energy level

1 2 3 4 5 6 7 8

A 3,500 calorie deficit will equal 1 lb of weight loss.

Notes/Journal

FOOD LOG

Day	Date	Week #

	Portion	Calories (kcal)	Fat (g)	Saturated Fat (g)	Sodium (mg)	Carbs (g)	Fiber (g)	Protein (g)	Other
BREAKFAST Time:									
Breakfast Totals →									
SNACK Time:									
Snack Totals →									
LUNCH Time:									
Lunch Totals →									
SNACK Time:									
Snack Totals →									
DINNER Time:									
Dinner Totals →									
SNACK Time:									
Snack Totals →									
Daily Totals →									

DAILY FOOD GOALS

target	actual	
		calories
		protein (g)
		carbs (g)
		fat (g)

water (8 oz glasses)

☐ ☐ ☐ ☐ ☐ ☐ ☐ ☐

fruits + vegetables (servings)

☐ ☐ ☐ ☐ ☐ ☐ ☐ ☐ ☐ ☐

FITNESS LOG

CARDIO/OTHER	Time of Day	Heart Rate	Duration	Speed	Level	Intensity	Other	Calories (kcal) Used
Calorie Totals								

WEIGHTS	Time of Day	Muscle Group	Reps	Sets	Duration	Intensity	Other	Calories (kcal) Used
Calorie Totals								

Total Calories Burned

Calories Consumed	−	Calories Used	=	Net Calories	−	BMR (Basal Metabolic Rate)	=	Net Calorie Deficit

Vitamins/Supplements	Dosage	Quantity

mood

☹ 2 3 4 5 6 7 ☺

energy level

1 2 3 4 5 6 7 8

A 3,500 calorie deficit will equal 1 lb of weight loss.

Notes/Journal

WEEKLY PROGRESS

	Weight	BMI	BMR	Heart Rate	Cholesterol	Blood Sugar	Other
STATS							
Last Week							
Current							

	Neck	Shoulder	Chest	Waist	Hip	Thigh	Calf	Arm	Other
MEASUREMENTS									
Last Week									
Current									

Notes/Journal

GOALS FOR NEXT WEEK

DAILY CALORIE DEFICIT

Day 1		Day 5	
Day 2		Day 6	
Day 3		Day 7	
Day 4		Weekly Total	

Waist Hip Ratio

Women <.7
Men   <.9

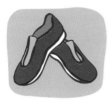

We are what we repeatedly do.
Excellence, then, is not an act, but a habit.

ARISTOTLE

TIP OF THE WEEK

Most important, wrap your mind around the idea that you need to be active for the rest of your life. Walking may melt off the weight you want to lose now, but if you stop moving once that extra heft's gone, it'll soon be back.

—Martica Heaner

FOOD LOG

Day	Date	Week #

	Portion	Calories (kcal)	Fat (g)	Saturated Fat (g)	Sodium (mg)	Carbs (g)	Fiber (g)	Protein (g)	Other
BREAKFAST Time:	Portion								
Breakfast Totals →									
SNACK Time:									
Snack Totals →									
LUNCH Time:									
Lunch Totals →									
SNACK Time:									
Snack Totals →									
DINNER Time:									
Dinner Totals →									
SNACK Time:									
Snack Totals →									
Daily Totals →									

DAILY FOOD GOALS

target	actual	
		calories
		protein (g)
		carbs (g)
		fat (g)

water (8 oz glasses)

☐ ☐ ☐ ☐ ☐ ☐ ☐ ☐

fruits + vegetables (servings)

☐ ☐ ☐ ☐ ☐ ☐ ☐ ☐ ☐

FITNESS LOG

CARDIO/OTHER	Time of Day	Heart Rate	Duration	Speed	Level	Intensity	Other	Calories (kcal) Used
Calorie Totals								

WEIGHTS	Time of Day	Muscle Group	Reps	Sets	Duration	Intensity	Other	Calories (kcal) Used
Calorie Totals								

Total Calories Burned

Calories Consumed	-	Calories Used	=	Net Calories	-	BMR (Basal Metabolic Rate)	=	Net Calorie Deficit

Vitamins/Supplements	Dosage	Quantity

mood

☹ 2 3 4 5 6 7 ☺

energy level

1 2 3 4 5 6 7 8

A 3,500 calorie deficit will equal 1 lb of weight loss.

Notes/Journal

FOOD LOG

	Day		Date		Week #

	Portion	Calories (kcal)	Fat (g)	Saturated Fat (g)	Sodium (mg)	Carbs (g)	Fiber (g)	Protein (g)	Other
BREAKFAST Time:									
Breakfast Totals →									
SNACK Time:									
Snack Totals →									
LUNCH Time:									
Lunch Totals →									
SNACK Time:									
Snack Totals →									
DINNER Time:									
Dinner Totals →									
SNACK Time:									
Snack Totals →									
Daily Totals →									

DAILY FOOD GOALS

target	actual	
		calories
		protein (g)
		carbs (g)
		fat (g)

water (8 oz glasses)

☐ ☐ ☐ ☐ ☐ ☐ ☐ ☐

fruits + vegetables (servings)

☐ ☐ ☐ ☐ ☐ ☐ ☐ ☐ ☐

FITNESS LOG

CARDIO/OTHER	Time of Day	Heart Rate	Duration	Speed	Level	Intensity	Other	Calories (kcal) Used
Calorie Totals								

WEIGHTS	Time of Day	Muscle Group	Reps	Sets	Duration	Intensity	Other	Calories (kcal) Used
Calorie Totals								
Total Calories Burned								

Calories Consumed	−	Calories Used	=	Net Calories	−	BMR (Basal Metabolic Rate)	=	Net Calorie Deficit

Vitamins/Supplements	Dosage	Quantity

mood

☹ 2 3 4 5 6 7 ☺

energy level

1 2 3 4 5 6 7 8

A 3,500 calorie deficit will equal 1 lb of weight loss.

Notes/Journal

FOOD LOG

| Day | | Date | | Week # |

	Portion	Calories (kcal)	Fat (g)	Saturated Fat (g)	Sodium (mg)	Carbs (g)	Fiber (g)	Protein (g)	Other
BREAKFAST Time:									
Breakfast Totals →									
SNACK Time:									
Snack Totals →									
LUNCH Time:									
Lunch Totals →									
SNACK Time:									
Snack Totals →									
DINNER Time:									
Dinner Totals →									
SNACK Time:									
Snack Totals →									
Daily Totals →									

DAILY FOOD GOALS

	target	actual	
			calories
			protein (g)
			carbs (g)
			fat (g)

water (8 oz glasses)

☐ ☐ ☐ ☐ ☐ ☐ ☐ ☐

fruits + vegetables (servings)

☐ ☐ ☐ ☐ ☐ ☐ ☐ ☐ ☐ ☐

FITNESS LOG

CARDIO/OTHER	Time of Day	Heart Rate	Duration	Speed	Level	Intensity	Other	Calories (kcal) Used
Calorie Totals								

WEIGHTS	Time of Day	Muscle Group	Reps	Sets	Duration	Intensity	Other	Calories (kcal) Used
Calorie Totals								

Total Calories Burned

Calories Consumed		Calories Used		Net Calories		BMR (Basal Metabolic Rate)		Net Calorie Deficit
	−		=		−		=	

Vitamins/Supplements	Dosage	Quantity

mood

☹ 2 3 4 5 6 7 ☺

energy level

1 2 3 4 5 6 7 8

A 3,500 calorie deficit will equal 1 lb of weight loss.

Notes/Journal

FOOD LOG

Day	Date	Week #

	Portion	Calories (kcal)	Fat (g)	Saturated Fat (g)	Sodium (mg)	Carbs (g)	Fiber (g)	Protein (g)	Othe
BREAKFAST Time:									
Breakfast Totals →									
SNACK Time:									
Snack Totals →									
LUNCH Time:									
Lunch Totals →									
SNACK Time:									
Snack Totals →									
DINNER Time:									
Dinner Totals →									
SNACK Time:									
Snack Totals →									
Daily Totals →									

DAILY FOOD GOALS

target	actual	
		calories
		protein (g)
		carbs (g)
		fat (g)

water (8 oz glasses)

☐ ☐ ☐ ☐ ☐ ☐ ☐ ☐ ☐

fruits + vegetables (servings)

☐ ☐ ☐ ☐ ☐ ☐ ☐ ☐ ☐ ☐ ☐

FITNESS LOG

CARDIO/OTHER	Time of Day	Heart Rate	Duration	Speed	Level	Intensity	Other	Calories (kcal) Used
Calorie Totals								

WEIGHTS	Time of Day	Muscle Group	Reps	Sets	Duration	Intensity	Other	Calories (kcal) Used
Calorie Totals								
Total Calories Burned								

Calories Consumed	−	Calories Used	=	Net Calories	−	BMR (Basal Metabolic Rate)	=	Net Calorie Deficit

Vitamins/Supplements	Dosage	Quantity

mood

☹ 2 3 4 5 6 7 ☺

energy level

1 2 3 4 5 6 7 8

A 3,500 calorie deficit will equal 1 lb of weight loss.

Notes/Journal

FOOD LOG

Day	Date	Week #

	Portion	Calories (kcal)	Fat (g)	Saturated Fat (g)	Sodium (mg)	Carbs (g)	Fiber (g)	Protein (g)	Other
BREAKFAST Time:									
Breakfast Totals →									
SNACK Time:									
Snack Totals →									
LUNCH Time:									
Lunch Totals →									
SNACK Time:									
Snack Totals →									
DINNER Time:									
Dinner Totals →									
SNACK Time:									
Snack Totals →									
Daily Totals →									

DAILY FOOD GOALS

target	actual	
		calories
		protein (g)
		carbs (g)
		fat (g)

water (8 oz glasses)

☐ ☐ ☐ ☐ ☐ ☐ ☐ ☐

fruits + vegetables (servings)

☐ ☐ ☐ ☐ ☐ ☐ ☐ ☐ ☐ ☐

FITNESS LOG

CARDIO/OTHER	Time of Day	Heart Rate	Duration	Speed	Level	Intensity	Other	Calories (kcal) Used
Calorie Totals								

WEIGHTS	Time of Day	Muscle Group	Reps	Sets	Duration	Intensity	Other	Calories (kcal) Used
Calorie Totals								

Total Calories Burned

Calories Consumed		Calories Used		Net Calories		BMR (Basal Metabolic Rate)		Net Calorie Deficit
	−		=		−		=	

Vitamins/Supplements	Dosage	Quantity		

mood

☹ 2 3 4 5 6 7 ☺

energy level

1 2 3 4 5 6 7 8

A 3,500 calorie deficit will equal 1 lb of weight loss.

Notes/Journal

FOOD LOG

Day	Date	Week #

	Calories (kcal)	Fat (g)	Saturated Fat (g)	Sodium (mg)	Carbs (g)	Fiber (g)	Protein (g)	Other
BREAKFAST Time: — Portion								
Breakfast Totals →								
SNACK Time:								
Snack Totals →								
LUNCH Time:								
Lunch Totals →								
SNACK Time:								
Snack Totals →								
DINNER Time:								
Dinner Totals →								
SNACK Time:								
Snack Totals →								
Daily Totals →								

DAILY FOOD GOALS

target	actual	
		calories
		protein (g)
		carbs (g)
		fat (g)

water (8 oz glasses)

☐ ☐ ☐ ☐ ☐ ☐ ☐ ☐

fruits + vegetables (servings)

☐ ☐ ☐ ☐ ☐ ☐ ☐ ☐ ☐

FITNESS LOG

CARDIO/OTHER	Time of Day	Heart Rate	Duration	Speed	Level	Intensity	Other	Calories (kcal) Used
Calorie Totals								

WEIGHTS	Time of Day	Muscle Group	Reps	Sets	Duration	Intensity	Other	Calories (kcal) Used
Calorie Totals								
Total Calories Burned								

Calories Consumed		Calories Used		Net Calories		BMR (Basal Metabolic Rate)		Net Calorie Deficit
	−		=		−		=	

Vitamins/Supplements	Dosage	Quantity

mood
☹ 2 3 4 5 6 7 ☺

energy level
1 2 3 4 5 6 7 8

A 3,500 calorie deficit will equal 1 lb of weight loss.

Notes/Journal

FOOD LOG

Day	Date	Week #

		Calories (kcal)	Fat (g)	Saturated Fat (g)	Sodium (mg)	Carbs (g)	Fiber (g)	Protein (g)	Other
BREAKFAST Time:	Portion								
Breakfast Totals →									
SNACK Time:									
Snack Totals →									
LUNCH Time:									
Lunch Totals →									
SNACK Time:									
Snack Totals →									
DINNER Time:									
Dinner Totals →									
SNACK Time:									
Snack Totals →									
Daily Totals →									

DAILY FOOD GOALS

target	actual	
		calories
		protein (g)
		carbs (g)
		fat (g)

water (8 oz glasses)

☐ ☐ ☐ ☐ ☐ ☐ ☐ ☐

fruits + vegetables (servings)

☐ ☐ ☐ ☐ ☐ ☐ ☐ ☐ ☐

FITNESS LOG

CARDIO/OTHER	Time of Day	Heart Rate	Duration	Speed	Level	Intensity	Other	Calories (kcal) Used
Calorie Totals								

WEIGHTS	Time of Day	Muscle Group	Reps	Sets	Duration	Intensity	Other	Calories (kcal) Used
Calorie Totals								

Total Calories Burned

Calories Consumed		Calories Used		Net Calories		BMR (Basal Metabolic Rate)		Net Calorie Deficit
	−		=		−		=	

Vitamins/Supplements	Dosage	Quantity	mood
			☹ 2 3 4 5 6 7 ☺
			energy level
			1 2 3 4 5 6 7 8

A 3,500 calorie deficit will equal 1 lb of weight loss.

Notes/Journal

WEEKLY PROGRESS

	Weight	BMI	BMR	Heart Rate	Cholesterol	Blood Sugar	Other
STATS							
Last Week							
Current							

	Neck	Shoulder	Chest	Waist	Hip	Thigh	Calf	Arm	Other
MEASUREMENTS									
Last Week									
Current									

Notes/Journal

GOALS FOR NEXT WEEK

DAILY CALORIE DEFICIT

Day 1		Day 5	
Day 2		Day 6	
Day 3		Day 7	
Day 4		Weekly Total	

Waist Hip Ratio

Women <.7
Men   <.9

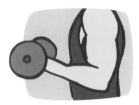

I learned something from all those sets and reps when I didn't think I could lift another ounce of weight. What I learned is that we are always stronger than we know.

Arnold Schwarzenegger

TIP OF THE WEEK

If your goal is to get stronger, strength-train first while your body is full of energy. You'll be able to lift more weight and do more repetitions. If you want to lose pounds, start with cardio. It raises your heart rate and boosts your calorie burn. Be sure to warm up for at least 5 to 10 minutes before you begin.

—Gary Scott

FOOD LOG

Day	Date	Week #

BREAKFAST Time:	Portion	Calories (kcal)	Fat (g)	Saturated Fat (g)	Sodium (mg)	Carbs (g)	Fiber (g)	Protein (g)	Other
Breakfast Totals →									
SNACK Time:									
Snack Totals →									
LUNCH Time:									
Lunch Totals →									
SNACK Time:									
Snack Totals →									
DINNER Time:									
Dinner Totals →									
SNACK Time:									
Snack Totals →									
Daily Totals →									

DAILY FOOD GOALS

	target	actual
calories		
protein (g)		
carbs (g)		
fat (g)		

water (8 oz glasses)

☐☐☐☐☐☐☐☐

fruits + vegetables (servings)

☐☐☐☐☐☐☐☐☐☐

FITNESS LOG

CARDIO/OTHER	Time of Day	Heart Rate	Duration	Speed	Level	Intensity	Other	Calories (kcal) Used

Calorie Totals

WEIGHTS	Time of Day	Muscle Group	Reps	Sets	Duration	Intensity	Other	Calories (kcal) Used

Calorie Totals

Total Calories Burned

Calories Consumed		Calories Used		Net Calories		BMR (Basal Metabolic Rate)		Net Calorie Deficit
	−		=		−		=	

Vitamins/Supplements	Dosage	Quantity

mood

☹ 2 3 4 5 6 7 ☺

energy level

1 2 3 4 5 6 7 8

A 3,500 calorie deficit will equal 1 lb of weight loss.

Notes/Journal

FOOD LOG

	Day	Date	Week #

	Portion	Calories (kcal)	Fat (g)	Saturated Fat (g)	Sodium (mg)	Carbs (g)	Fiber (g)	Protein (g)	Other
BREAKFAST Time:									
Breakfast Totals →									
SNACK Time:									
Snack Totals →									
LUNCH Time:									
Lunch Totals →									
SNACK Time:									
Snack Totals →									
DINNER Time:									
Dinner Totals →									
SNACK Time:									
Snack Totals →									
Daily Totals →									

DAILY FOOD GOALS

target	actual	
		calories
		protein (g)
		carbs (g)
		fat (g)

water (8 oz glasses)

☐ ☐ ☐ ☐ ☐ ☐ ☐ ☐

fruits + vegetables (servings)

☐ ☐ ☐ ☐ ☐ ☐ ☐ ☐ ☐ ☐

FITNESS LOG

CARDIO/OTHER	Time of Day	Heart Rate	Duration	Speed	Level	Intensity	Other	Calories (kcal) Used
Calorie Totals								

WEIGHTS	Time of Day	Muscle Group	Reps	Sets	Duration	Intensity	Other	Calories (kcal) Used
Calorie Totals								
Total Calories Burned								

Calories Consumed		Calories Used		Net Calories		BMR (Basal Metabolic Rate)		Net Calorie Deficit
	−		=		−		=	

Vitamins/Supplements	Dosage	Quantity

mood

☹ 2 3 4 5 6 7 ☺

energy level

1 2 3 4 5 6 7 8

A 3,500 calorie deficit will equal 1 lb of weight loss.

Notes/Journal

FOOD LOG

Day	Date	Week #

	Portion	Calories (kcal)	Fat (g)	Saturated Fat (g)	Sodium (mg)	Carbs (g)	Fiber (g)	Protein (g)	Other
BREAKFAST Time:									
Breakfast Totals →									
SNACK Time:									
Snack Totals →									
LUNCH Time:									
Lunch Totals →									
SNACK Time:									
Snack Totals →									
DINNER Time:									
Dinner Totals →									
SNACK Time:									
Snack Totals →									
Daily Totals →									

DAILY FOOD GOALS

target	actual	
		calories
		protein (g)
		carbs (g)
		fat (g)

water (8 oz glasses)

☐☐☐☐☐☐☐☐

fruits + vegetables (servings)

☐☐☐☐☐☐☐☐☐

FITNESS LOG

CARDIO/OTHER	Time of Day	Heart Rate	Duration	Speed	Level	Intensity	Other	Calories (kcal) Used
Calorie Totals								

WEIGHTS	Time of Day	Muscle Group	Reps	Sets	Duration	Intensity	Other	Calories (kcal) Used
Calorie Totals								

Total Calories Burned

Calories Consumed	−	Calories Used	=	Net Calories	−	BMR (Basal Metabolic Rate)	=	Net Calorie Deficit

Vitamins/Supplements	Dosage	Quantity

mood

☹ 2 3 4 5 6 7 ☺

energy level

1 2 3 4 5 6 7 8

A 3,500 calorie deficit will equal 1 lb of weight loss.

Notes/Journal

FOOD LOG

Day	Date	Week #

	Portion	Calories (kcal)	Fat (g)	Saturated Fat (g)	Sodium (mg)	Carbs (g)	Fiber (g)	Protein (g)	Other
BREAKFAST Time:									
Breakfast Totals →									
SNACK Time:									
Snack Totals →									
LUNCH Time:									
Lunch Totals →									
SNACK Time:									
Snack Totals →									
DINNER Time:									
Dinner Totals →									
SNACK Time:									
Snack Totals →									
Daily Totals →									

DAILY FOOD GOALS

target	actual	
		calories
		protein (g)
		carbs (g)
		fat (g)

water (8 oz glasses)

☐ ☐ ☐ ☐ ☐ ☐ ☐ ☐

fruits + vegetables (servings)

☐ ☐ ☐ ☐ ☐ ☐ ☐ ☐ ☐

FITNESS LOG

CARDIO/OTHER	Time of Day	Heart Rate	Duration	Speed	Level	Intensity	Other	Calories (kcal) Used
Calorie Totals								

WEIGHTS	Time of Day	Muscle Group	Reps	Sets	Duration	Intensity	Other	Calories (kcal) Used
Calorie Totals								

Total Calories Burned

Calories Consumed	−	Calories Used	=	Net Calories	−	BMR (Basal Metabolic Rate)	=	Net Calorie Deficit

Vitamins/Supplements	Dosage	Quantity

mood

☹ 2 3 4 5 6 7 ☺

energy level

1 2 3 4 5 6 7 8

A 3,500 calorie deficit will equal 1 lb of weight loss.

Notes/Journal

FOOD LOG

Day	Date	Week #

		Portion	Calories (kcal)	Fat (g)	Saturated Fat (g)	Sodium (mg)	Carbs (g)	Fiber (g)	Protein (g)	Other
BREAKFAST Time:										
Breakfast Totals →										
SNACK Time:										
Snack Totals →										
LUNCH Time:										
Lunch Totals →										
SNACK Time:										
Snack Totals →										
DINNER Time:										
Dinner Totals →										
SNACK Time:										
Snack Totals →										
Daily Totals →										

DAILY FOOD GOALS

target	actual	
		calories
		protein (g)
		carbs (g)
		fat (g)

water (8 oz glasses)

☐ ☐ ☐ ☐ ☐ ☐ ☐ ☐

fruits + vegetables (servings)

☐ ☐ ☐ ☐ ☐ ☐ ☐ ☐ ☐

FITNESS LOG

CARDIO/OTHER	Time of Day	Heart Rate	Duration	Speed	Level	Intensity	Other	Calories (kcal) Used
Calorie Totals								

WEIGHTS	Time of Day	Muscle Group	Reps	Sets	Duration	Intensity	Other	Calories (kcal) Used
Calorie Totals								
Total Calories Burned								

Calories Consumed	−	Calories Used	=	Net Calories	−	BMR (Basal Metabolic Rate)	=	Net Calorie Deficit

Vitamins/Supplements	Dosage	Quantity

mood

☹ 2 3 4 5 6 7 ☺

energy level

1 2 3 4 5 6 7 8

A 3,500 calorie deficit will equal 1 lb of weight loss.

Notes/Journal

FOOD LOG

		Day		Date			Week #

	Portion	Calories (kcal)	Fat (g)	Saturated Fat (g)	Sodium (mg)	Carbs (g)	Fiber (g)	Protein (g)	Other
BREAKFAST Time:									
Breakfast Totals →									
SNACK Time:									
Snack Totals →									
LUNCH Time:									
Lunch Totals →									
SNACK Time:									
Snack Totals →									
DINNER Time:									
Dinner Totals →									
SNACK Time:									
Snack Totals →									
Daily Totals →									

DAILY FOOD GOALS

	target	actual
calories		
protein (g)		
carbs (g)		
fat (g)		

water (8 oz glasses)

☐ ☐ ☐ ☐ ☐ ☐ ☐ ☐

fruits + vegetables (servings)

☐ ☐ ☐ ☐ ☐ ☐ ☐ ☐ ☐

FITNESS LOG

CARDIO/OTHER	Time of Day	Heart Rate	Duration	Speed	Level	Intensity	Other	Calories (kcal) Used
Calorie Totals								

WEIGHTS	Time of Day	Muscle Group	Reps	Sets	Duration	Intensity	Other	Calories (kcal) Used
Calorie Totals								

Total Calories Burned

Calories Consumed	-	Calories Used	=	Net Calories	-	BMR (Basal Metabolic Rate)	=	Net Calorie Deficit

Vitamins/Supplements	Dosage	Quantity

mood

☹ 2 3 4 5 6 7 ☺

energy level

1 2 3 4 5 6 7 8

A 3,500 calorie deficit will equal 1 lb of weight loss.

Notes/Journal

FOOD LOG

Day		Date		Week #

	Portion	Calories (kcal)	Fat (g)	Saturated Fat (g)	Sodium (mg)	Carbs (g)	Fiber (g)	Protein (g)	Other*
BREAKFAST Time:									
Breakfast Totals →									
SNACK Time:									
Snack Totals →									
LUNCH Time:									
Lunch Totals →									
SNACK Time:									
Snack Totals →									
DINNER Time:									
Dinner Totals →									
SNACK Time:									
Snack Totals →									
Daily Totals →									

DAILY FOOD GOALS

target	actual	
		calories
		protein (g)
		carbs (g)
		fat (g)

water (8 oz glasses)

☐ ☐ ☐ ☐ ☐ ☐ ☐ ☐

fruits + vegetables (servings)

☐ ☐ ☐ ☐ ☐ ☐ ☐ ☐ ☐ ☐

FITNESS LOG

CARDIO/OTHER	Time of Day	Heart Rate	Duration	Speed	Level	Intensity	Other	Calories (kcal) Used
Calorie Totals								

WEIGHTS	Time of Day	Muscle Group	Reps	Sets	Duration	Intensity	Other	Calories (kcal) Used
Calorie Totals								
Total Calories Burned								

Calories Consumed		Calories Used		Net Calories		BMR (Basal Metabolic Rate)		Net Calorie Deficit
	-		=		-		=	

Vitamins/Supplements	Dosage	Quantity

mood

☹ 2 3 4 5 6 7 ☺

energy level

1 2 3 4 5 6 7 8

A 3,500 calorie deficit will equal 1 lb of weight loss.

Notes/Journal

WEEKLY PROGRESS

STATS	Weight	BMI	BMR	Heart Rate	Cholesterol	Blood Sugar	Other
Last Week							
Current							

MEASUREMENTS	Neck	Shoulder	Chest	Waist	Hip	Thigh	Calf	Arm	Other
Last Week									
Current									

Notes/Journal

GOALS FOR NEXT WEEK

DAILY CALORIE DEFICIT

Day 1		Day 5	
Day 2		Day 6	
Day 3		Day 7	
Day 4		Weekly Total	

Waist Hip Ratio

Women <.7
Men   <.9

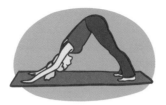

Body care is an exercise in sensibility.
Get enough sleep. Nurture yourself with
healthful foods. Exercise in a way you enjoy
enough to do regularly—start off the day with
your own private dance party, for instance.
Stretch like a cat whenever you get up.
And don't forget to breathe.

BARBARA PAULDING

TIP OF THE WEEK

Stress response, whether it is "fight-or-flight," juggling too many responsibilities, or coping with financial pressures, triggers a biochemical process where our bodies go into survival mode. Our bodies store fuel, slow down metabolism, and dump out chemicals [cortisol, leptin, and other hormones] which are more likely to cause . . . obesity in the abdominal region.

—Michelle May

FOOD LOG

Day		Date		Week #	

	Portion	Calories (kcal)	Fat (g)	Saturated Fat (g)	Sodium (mg)	Carbs (g)	Fiber (g)	Protein (g)	Other
BREAKFAST Time:	Portion								
Breakfast Totals →									
SNACK Time:									
Snack Totals →									
LUNCH Time:									
Lunch Totals →									
SNACK Time:									
Snack Totals →									
DINNER Time:									
Dinner Totals →									
SNACK Time:									
Snack Totals →									
Daily Totals →									

DAILY FOOD GOALS

	target	actual	
			calories
			protein (g)
			carbs (g)
			fat (g)

water (8 oz glasses)

☐☐☐☐☐☐☐☐☐

fruits + vegetables (servings)

☐☐☐☐☐☐☐☐☐☐

FITNESS LOG

CARDIO/OTHER	Time of Day	Heart Rate	Duration	Speed	Level	Intensity	Other	Calories (kcal) Used
Calorie Totals								

WEIGHTS	Time of Day	Muscle Group	Reps	Sets	Duration	Intensity	Other	Calories (kcal) Used
Calorie Totals								
Total Calories Burned								

Calories Consumed		Calories Used		Net Calories		BMR (Basal Metabolic Rate)		Net Calorie Deficit
	−		=		−		=	

Vitamins/Supplements	Dosage	Quantity

mood

☹ 2 3 4 5 6 7 ☺

energy level

1 2 3 4 5 6 7 8

A 3,500 calorie deficit will equal 1 lb of weight loss.

Notes/Journal

FOOD LOG

Day	Date	Week #

	Portion	Calories (kcal)	Fat (g)	Saturated Fat (g)	Sodium (mg)	Carbs (g)	Fiber (g)	Protein (g)	Other
BREAKFAST Time:									
Breakfast Totals →									
SNACK Time:									
Snack Totals →									
LUNCH Time:									
Lunch Totals →									
SNACK Time:									
Snack Totals →									
DINNER Time:									
Dinner Totals →									
SNACK Time:									
Snack Totals →									
Daily Totals →									

DAILY FOOD GOALS

target	actual	
		calories
		protein (g)
		carbs (g)
		fat (g)

water (8 oz glasses)

☐☐☐☐☐☐☐☐

fruits + vegetables (servings)

☐☐☐☐☐☐☐☐☐

FITNESS LOG

CARDIO/OTHER	Time of Day	Heart Rate	Duration	Speed	Level	Intensity	Other	Calories (kcal) Used
Calorie Totals								

WEIGHTS	Time of Day	Muscle Group	Reps	Sets	Duration	Intensity	Other	Calories (kcal) Used
Calorie Totals								
Total Calories Burned								

Calories Consumed − Calories Used = Net Calories − BMR (Basal Metabolic Rate) = Net Calorie Deficit

Vitamins/Supplements	Dosage	Quantity

mood

☹ 2 3 4 5 6 7 ☺

energy level

1 2 3 4 5 6 7 8

A 3,500 calorie deficit will equal 1 lb of weight loss.

Notes/Journal

FOOD LOG

	Day	Date	Week #

	Portion	Calories (kcal)	Fat (g)	Saturated Fat (g)	Sodium (mg)	Carbs (g)	Fiber (g)	Protein (g)	Other
BREAKFAST Time:									
Breakfast Totals →									
SNACK Time:									
Snack Totals →									
LUNCH Time:									
Lunch Totals →									
SNACK Time:									
Snack Totals →									
DINNER Time:									
Dinner Totals →									
SNACK Time:									
Snack Totals →									
Daily Totals →									

DAILY FOOD GOALS

	target	actual
calories		
protein (g)		
carbs (g)		
fat (g)		

water (8 oz glasses)

☐ ☐ ☐ ☐ ☐ ☐ ☐ ☐

fruits + vegetables (servings)

☐ ☐ ☐ ☐ ☐ ☐ ☐ ☐ ☐

FITNESS LOG

CARDIO/OTHER	Time of Day	Heart Rate	Duration	Speed	Level	Intensity	Other	Calories (kcal) Used
Calorie Totals								

WEIGHTS	Time of Day	Muscle Group	Reps	Sets	Duration	Intensity	Other	Calories (kcal) Used
Calorie Totals								

Total Calories Burned

Calories Consumed	−	Calories Used	=	Net Calories	−	BMR (Basal Metabolic Rate)	=	Net Calorie Deficit

Vitamins/Supplements	Dosage	Quantity

mood

☹ 2 3 4 5 6 7 ☺

energy level

1 2 3 4 5 6 7 8

A 3,500 calorie deficit will equal 1 lb of weight loss.

Notes/Journal

FOOD LOG

Day	Date	Week #

			Calories (kcal)	Fat (g)	Saturated Fat (g)	Sodium (mg)	Carbs (g)	Fiber (g)	Protein (g)	Other
BREAKFAST Time:		Portion								
Breakfast Totals →										
SNACK Time:										
Snack Totals →										
LUNCH Time:										
Lunch Totals →										
SNACK Time:										
Snack Totals →										
DINNER Time:										
Dinner Totals →										
SNACK Time:										
Snack Totals →										
Daily Totals →										

DAILY FOOD GOALS

	target	actual
calories		
protein (g)		
carbs (g)		
fat (g)		

water (8 oz glasses)

☐ ☐ ☐ ☐ ☐ ☐ ☐ ☐

fruits + vegetables (servings)

☐ ☐ ☐ ☐ ☐ ☐ ☐ ☐ ☐ ☐

FITNESS LOG

CARDIO/OTHER	Time of Day	Heart Rate	Duration	Speed	Level	Intensity	Other	Calories (kcal) Used
Calorie Totals								

WEIGHTS	Time of Day	Muscle Group	Reps	Sets	Duration	Intensity	Other	Calories (kcal) Used
Calorie Totals								
Total Calories Burned								

Calories Consumed	−	Calories Used	=	Net Calories	−	BMR (Basal Metabolic Rate)	=	Net Calorie Deficit

Vitamins/Supplements	Dosage	Quantity

mood

☹ 2 3 4 5 6 7 ☺

energy level

1 2 3 4 5 6 7 8

A 3,500 calorie deficit will equal 1 lb of weight loss.

Notes/Journal

FOOD LOG

Day	Date	Week #

		Calories (kcal)	Fat (g)	Saturated Fat (g)	Sodium (mg)	Carbs (g)	Fiber (g)	Protein (g)	Other
BREAKFAST Time:	Portion								
Breakfast Totals →									
SNACK Time:									
Snack Totals →									
LUNCH Time:									
Lunch Totals →									
SNACK Time:									
Snack Totals →									
DINNER Time:									
Dinner Totals →									
SNACK Time:									
Snack Totals →									
Daily Totals →									

DAILY FOOD GOALS

target	actual	
		calories
		protein (g)
		carbs (g)
		fat (g)

water (8 oz glasses)

☐ ☐ ☐ ☐ ☐ ☐ ☐ ☐

fruits + vegetables (servings)

☐ ☐ ☐ ☐ ☐ ☐ ☐ ☐ ☐

FITNESS LOG

CARDIO/OTHER	Time of Day	Heart Rate	Duration	Speed	Level	Intensity	Other	Calories (kcal) Used
Calorie Totals								

WEIGHTS	Time of Day	Muscle Group	Reps	Sets	Duration	Intensity	Other	Calories (kcal) Used
Calorie Totals								

Total Calories Burned

Calories Consumed	−	Calories Used	=	Net Calories	−	BMR (Basal Metabolic Rate)	=	Net Calorie Deficit

Vitamins/Supplements	Dosage	Quantity

mood

☹ 2 3 4 5 6 7 ☺

energy level

1 2 3 4 5 6 7 8

A 3,500 calorie deficit will equal 1 lb of weight loss.

Notes/Journal

FOOD LOG	Day		Date		Week #	

		Calories (kcal)	Fat (g)	Saturated Fat (g)	Sodium (mg)	Carbs (g)	Fiber (g)	Protein (g)	Othe
BREAKFAST Time:	Portion								
Breakfast Totals →									
SNACK Time:									
Snack Totals →									
LUNCH Time:									
Lunch Totals →									
SNACK Time:									
Snack Totals →									
DINNER Time:									
Dinner Totals →									
SNACK Time:									
Snack Totals →									
Daily Totals →									

DAILY FOOD GOALS

target	actual	
		calories
		protein (g)
		carbs (g)
		fat (g)

water (8 oz glasses)

☐ ☐ ☐ ☐ ☐ ☐ ☐ ☐

fruits + vegetables (servings)

☐ ☐ ☐ ☐ ☐ ☐ ☐ ☐ ☐ ☐

FITNESS LOG

CARDIO/OTHER	Time of Day	Heart Rate	Duration	Speed	Level	Intensity	Other	Calories (kcal) Used
Calorie Totals								

WEIGHTS	Time of Day	Muscle Group	Reps	Sets	Duration	Intensity	Other	Calories (kcal) Used
Calorie Totals								

Total Calories Burned

Calories Consumed	−	Calories Used	=	Net Calories	−	BMR (Basal Metabolic Rate)	=	Net Calorie Deficit

Vitamins/Supplements	Dosage	Quantity

mood

☹ 2 3 4 5 6 7 ☺

energy level

1 2 3 4 5 6 7 8

A 3,500 calorie deficit will equal 1 lb of weight loss.

Notes/Journal

FOOD LOG

	Day	Date	Week #

	Portion	Calories (kcal)	Fat (g)	Saturated Fat (g)	Sodium (mg)	Carbs (g)	Fiber (g)	Protein (g)	Other
BREAKFAST Time:									
Breakfast Totals →									
SNACK Time:									
Snack Totals →									
LUNCH Time:									
Lunch Totals →									
SNACK Time:									
Snack Totals →									
DINNER Time:									
Dinner Totals →									
SNACK Time:									
Snack Totals →									
Daily Totals →									

DAILY FOOD GOALS

target	actual	
		calories
		protein (g)
		carbs (g)
		fat (g)

water (8 oz glasses)

☐ ☐ ☐ ☐ ☐ ☐ ☐ ☐

fruits + vegetables (servings)

☐ ☐ ☐ ☐ ☐ ☐ ☐ ☐ ☐

FITNESS LOG

CARDIO/OTHER	Time of Day	Heart Rate	Duration	Speed	Level	Intensity	Other	Calories (kcal) Used
Calorie Totals								

WEIGHTS	Time of Day	Muscle Group	Reps	Sets	Duration	Intensity	Other	Calories (kcal) Used
Calorie Totals								

Total Calories Burned

Calories Consumed - Calories Used = Net Calories - BMR (Basal Metabolic Rate) = Net Calorie Deficit

Vitamins/Supplements	Dosage	Quantity

mood

☹ 2 3 4 5 6 7 ☺

energy level

1 2 3 4 5 6 7 8

A 3,500 calorie deficit will equal 1 lb of weight loss.

Notes/Journal

WEEKLY PROGRESS

	Weight	BMI	BMR	Heart Rate	Cholesterol	Blood Sugar	Other
STATS							
Last Week							
Current							

	Neck	Shoulder	Chest	Waist	Hip	Thigh	Calf	Arm	Other
MEASUREMENTS									
Last Week									
Current									

Notes/Journal

_____
_____
_____
_____
_____
_____
_____
_____
_____
_____

GOALS FOR NEXT WEEK

_____
_____
_____
_____
_____
_____
_____
_____

DAILY CALORIE DEFICIT

Day 1		Day 5	
Day 2		Day 6	
Day 3		Day 7	
Day 4		Weekly Total	

Waist Hip Ratio
Women <.7
Men   <.9

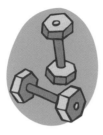

Lack of activity destroys the good condition of every human being, while movement and methodical physical exercise save it and preserve it.

PLATO

TIP OF THE WEEK

Research has proven that two short bouts of exercise per day will actually stimulate the metabolism more than one longer bout. Go for a brisk 15-minute walk first thing in the morning before work and then another one at lunch time. Do this 5 days per week and I know you'll see progress at the end of 30 days.

—Raphael Calzadilla

FOOD LOG

Day	Date	Week #

		Calories (kcal)	Fat (g)	Saturated Fat (g)	Sodium (mg)	Carbs (g)	Fiber (g)	Protein (g)	Other
BREAKFAST Time:	Portion								
Breakfast Totals →									
SNACK Time:									
Snack Totals →									
LUNCH Time:									
Lunch Totals →									
SNACK Time:									
Snack Totals →									
DINNER Time:									
Dinner Totals →									
SNACK Time:									
Snack Totals →									
Daily Totals →									

DAILY FOOD GOALS

target	actual	
		calories
		protein (g)
		carbs (g)
		fat (g)

water (8 oz glasses)

☐ ☐ ☐ ☐ ☐ ☐ ☐ ☐

fruits + vegetables (servings)

☐ ☐ ☐ ☐ ☐ ☐ ☐ ☐ ☐ ☐

FITNESS LOG

CARDIO/OTHER	Time of Day	Heart Rate	Duration	Speed	Level	Intensity	Other	Calories (kcal) Used
Calorie Totals								

WEIGHTS	Time of Day	Muscle Group	Reps	Sets	Duration	Intensity	Other	Calories (kcal) Used
Calorie Totals								

Total Calories Burned

Calories Consumed	−	Calories Used	=	Net Calories	−	BMR (Basal Metabolic Rate)	=	Net Calorie Deficit

Vitamins/Supplements	Dosage	Quantity

mood

☹ 2 3 4 5 6 7 ☺

energy level

1 2 3 4 5 6 7 8

A 3,500 calorie deficit will equal 1 lb of weight loss.

Notes/Journal

FOOD LOG

	Day	Date	Week #

	Portion	Calories (kcal)	Fat (g)	Saturated Fat (g)	Sodium (mg)	Carbs (g)	Fiber (g)	Protein (g)	Other
BREAKFAST Time:									
Breakfast Totals →									
SNACK Time:									
Snack Totals →									
LUNCH Time:									
Lunch Totals →									
SNACK Time:									
Snack Totals →									
DINNER Time:									
Dinner Totals →									
SNACK Time:									
Snack Totals →									
Daily Totals →									

DAILY FOOD GOALS

target	actual	
		calories
		protein (g)
		carbs (g)
		fat (g)

water (8 oz glasses)

☐ ☐ ☐ ☐ ☐ ☐ ☐ ☐

fruits + vegetables (servings)

☐ ☐ ☐ ☐ ☐ ☐ ☐ ☐ ☐

FITNESS LOG

CARDIO/OTHER	Time of Day	Heart Rate	Duration	Speed	Level	Intensity	Other	Calories (kcal) Used
Calorie Totals								

WEIGHTS	Time of Day	Muscle Group	Reps	Sets	Duration	Intensity	Other	Calories (kcal) Used
Calorie Totals								

Total Calories Burned

Calories Consumed	-	Calories Used	=	Net Calories	-	BMR (Basal Metabolic Rate)	=	Net Calorie Deficit

Vitamins/Supplements	Dosage	Quantity

mood

😞 2 3 4 5 6 7 😊

energy level

1 2 3 4 5 6 7 8

A 3,500 calorie deficit will equal 1 lb of weight loss.

Notes/Journal

FOOD LOG

	Day	Date	Week #

	Portion	Calories (kcal)	Fat (g)	Saturated Fat (g)	Sodium (mg)	Carbs (g)	Fiber (g)	Protein (g)	Other
BREAKFAST Time:									
Breakfast Totals →									
SNACK Time:									
Snack Totals →									
LUNCH Time:									
Lunch Totals →									
SNACK Time:									
Snack Totals →									
DINNER Time:									
Dinner Totals →									
SNACK Time:									
Snack Totals →									
Daily Totals →									

DAILY FOOD GOALS

target	actual	
		calories
		protein (g)
		carbs (g)
		fat (g)

water (8 oz glasses)

☐☐☐☐☐☐☐☐

fruits + vegetables (servings)

☐☐☐☐☐☐☐☐☐☐

FITNESS LOG

CARDIO/OTHER	Time of Day	Heart Rate	Duration	Speed	Level	Intensity	Other	Calories (kcal) Used
Calorie Totals								

WEIGHTS	Time of Day	Muscle Group	Reps	Sets	Duration	Intensity	Other	Calories (kcal) Used
Calorie Totals								

Total Calories Burned

Calories Consumed	−	Calories Used	=	Net Calories	−	BMR (Basal Metabolic Rate)	=	Net Calorie Deficit

Vitamins/Supplements	Dosage	Quantity

mood

☹ 2 3 4 5 6 7 ☺

energy level

1 2 3 4 5 6 7 8

A 3,500 calorie deficit will equal 1 lb of weight loss.

Notes/Journal

FOOD LOG

		Day		Date		Week #	

	Portion	Calories (kcal)	Fat (g)	Saturated Fat (g)	Sodium (mg)	Carbs (g)	Fiber (g)	Protein (g)	Other
BREAKFAST Time:									
Breakfast Totals →									
SNACK Time:									
Snack Totals →									
LUNCH Time:									
Lunch Totals →									
SNACK Time:									
Snack Totals →									
DINNER Time:									
Dinner Totals →									
SNACK Time:									
Snack Totals →									
Daily Totals →									

DAILY FOOD GOALS

	target	actual
calories		
protein (g)		
carbs (g)		
fat (g)		

water (8 oz glasses)

☐ ☐ ☐ ☐ ☐ ☐ ☐ ☐

fruits + vegetables (servings)

☐ ☐ ☐ ☐ ☐ ☐ ☐ ☐ ☐

FITNESS LOG

CARDIO/OTHER	Time of Day	Heart Rate	Duration	Speed	Level	Intensity	Other	Calories (kcal) Used
Calorie Totals								

WEIGHTS	Time of Day	Muscle Group	Reps	Sets	Duration	Intensity	Other	Calories (kcal) Used
Calorie Totals								
Total Calories Burned								

Calories Consumed	–	Calories Used	=	Net Calories	–	BMR (Basal Metabolic Rate)	=	Net Calorie Deficit

Vitamins/Supplements	Dosage	Quantity

mood

☹ 2 3 4 5 6 7 ☺

energy level

1 2 3 4 5 6 7 8

A 3,500 calorie deficit will equal 1 lb of weight loss.

Notes/Journal

FOOD LOG

Day	Date	Week #

	Portion	Calories (kcal)	Fat (g)	Saturated Fat (g)	Sodium (mg)	Carbs (g)	Fiber (g)	Protein (g)	Other
BREAKFAST Time:									
Breakfast Totals →									
SNACK Time:									
Snack Totals →									
LUNCH Time:									
Lunch Totals →									
SNACK Time:									
Snack Totals →									
DINNER Time:									
Dinner Totals →									
SNACK Time:									
Snack Totals →									
Daily Totals →									

DAILY FOOD GOALS

	target	actual	
			calories
			protein (g)
			carbs (g)
			fat (g)

water (8 oz glasses)

☐ ☐ ☐ ☐ ☐ ☐ ☐ ☐

fruits + vegetables (servings)

☐ ☐ ☐ ☐ ☐ ☐ ☐ ☐ ☐ ☐

FITNESS LOG

CARDIO/OTHER	Time of Day	Heart Rate	Duration	Speed	Level	Intensity	Other	Calories (kcal) Used
Calorie Totals								

WEIGHTS	Time of Day	Muscle Group	Reps	Sets	Duration	Intensity	Other	Calories (kcal) Used
Calorie Totals								

Total Calories Burned

Calories Consumed	-	Calories Used	=	Net Calories	-	BMR (Basal Metabolic Rate)	=	Net Calorie Deficit

Vitamins/Supplements	Dosage	Quantity

mood

☹ 2 3 4 5 6 7 ☺

energy level

1 2 3 4 5 6 7 8

A 3,500 calorie deficit will equal 1 lb of weight loss.

Notes/Journal

FOOD LOG

Day	Date	Week #

	Portion	Calories (kcal)	Fat (g)	Saturated Fat (g)	Sodium (mg)	Carbs (g)	Fiber (g)	Protein (g)	Other
BREAKFAST Time:									
Breakfast Totals →									
SNACK Time:									
Snack Totals →									
LUNCH Time:									
Lunch Totals →									
SNACK Time:									
Snack Totals →									
DINNER Time:									
Dinner Totals →									
SNACK Time:									
Snack Totals →									
Daily Totals →									

DAILY FOOD GOALS

target	actual	
		calories
		protein (g)
		carbs (g)
		fat (g)

water (8 oz glasses)
☐ ☐ ☐ ☐ ☐ ☐ ☐ ☐ ☐

fruits + vegetables (servings)
☐ ☐ ☐ ☐ ☐ ☐ ☐ ☐ ☐ ☐

FITNESS LOG

CARDIO/OTHER	Time of Day	Heart Rate	Duration	Speed	Level	Intensity	Other	Calories (kcal) Used
Calorie Totals								

WEIGHTS	Time of Day	Muscle Group	Reps	Sets	Duration	Intensity	Other	Calories (kcal) Used
Calorie Totals								
Total Calories Burned								

Calories Consumed	−	Calories Used	=	Net Calories	−	BMR (Basal Metabolic Rate)	=	Net Calorie Deficit

Vitamins/Supplements	Dosage	Quantity

mood
☹ 2 3 4 5 6 7 ☺

energy level
1 2 3 4 5 6 7 8

A 3,500 calorie deficit will equal 1 lb of weight loss.

Notes/Journal

FOOD LOG	Day	Date	Week #

	Portion	Calories (kcal)	Fat (g)	Saturated Fat (g)	Sodium (mg)	Carbs (g)	Fiber (g)	Protein (g)	Other
BREAKFAST Time:									
Breakfast Totals →									
SNACK Time:									
Snack Totals →									
LUNCH Time:									
Lunch Totals →									
SNACK Time:									
Snack Totals →									
DINNER Time:									
Dinner Totals →									
SNACK Time:									
Snack Totals →									
Daily Totals →									

DAILY FOOD GOALS

target	actual	
		calories
		protein (g)
		carbs (g)
		fat (g)

water (8 oz glasses)

☐☐☐☐☐☐☐☐

fruits + vegetables (servings)

☐☐☐☐☐☐☐☐☐☐

FITNESS LOG

CARDIO/OTHER	Time of Day	Heart Rate	Duration	Speed	Level	Intensity	Other	Calories (kcal) Used
Calorie Totals								

WEIGHTS	Time of Day	Muscle Group	Reps	Sets	Duration	Intensity	Other	Calories (kcal) Used
Calorie Totals								

Total Calories Burned

Calories Consumed	−	Calories Used	=	Net Calories	−	BMR (Basal Metabolic Rate)	=	Net Calorie Deficit

Vitamins/Supplements	Dosage	Quantity

mood

☹ 2 3 4 5 6 7 ☺

energy level

1 2 3 4 5 6 7 8

A 3,500 calorie deficit will equal 1 lb of weight loss.

Notes/Journal

WEEKLY PROGRESS

STATS	Weight	BMI	BMR	Heart Rate	Cholesterol	Blood Sugar	Other
Last Week							
Current							

MEASUREMENTS	Neck	Shoulder	Chest	Waist	Hip	Thigh	Calf	Arm	Other
Last Week									
Current									

Notes/Journal

GOALS FOR NEXT WEEK

DAILY CALORIE DEFICIT

Day 1		Day 5	
Day 2		Day 6	
Day 3		Day 7	
Day 4		Weekly Total	

Waist Hip Ratio

Women <.7
Men   <.9

A sound mind in a sound body is a short but full description of a happy state in this world.

JOHN LOCKE

TIP OF THE WEEK

If you are active, you cannot live, breathe, and think on 1,000 calories per day. Your body will not function properly and anything extra you put in your body will be stored as body fat, as you are in a state of famine. You need to regulate your calories by your daily activities. More activity equals more calories.

—Allison Ethier

FOOD LOG

Day	Date	Week #

	Portion	Calories (kcal)	Fat (g)	Saturated Fat (g)	Sodium (mg)	Carbs (g)	Fiber (g)	Protein (g)	Other
BREAKFAST Time:									
Breakfast Totals →									
SNACK Time:									
Snack Totals →									
LUNCH Time:									
Lunch Totals →									
SNACK Time:									
Snack Totals →									
DINNER Time:									
Dinner Totals →									
SNACK Time:									
Snack Totals →									
Daily Totals →									

DAILY FOOD GOALS

target	actual	
		calories
		protein (g)
		carbs (g)
		fat (g)

water (8 oz glasses)

☐ ☐ ☐ ☐ ☐ ☐ ☐ ☐

fruits + vegetables (servings)

☐ ☐ ☐ ☐ ☐ ☐ ☐ ☐ ☐ ☐

FITNESS LOG

CARDIO/OTHER	Time of Day	Heart Rate	Duration	Speed	Level	Intensity	Other	Calories (kcal) Used
Calorie Totals								

WEIGHTS	Time of Day	Muscle Group	Reps	Sets	Duration	Intensity	Other	Calories (kcal) Used
Calorie Totals								

Total Calories Burned

Calories Consumed	−	Calories Used	=	Net Calories	−	BMR (Basal Metabolic Rate)	=	Net Calorie Deficit

Vitamins/Supplements	Dosage	Quantity

mood

☹ 2 3 4 5 6 7 ☺

energy level

1 2 3 4 5 6 7 8

A 3,500 calorie deficit will equal 1 lb of weight loss.

Notes/Journal

FOOD LOG

Day	Date	Week #

		Calories (kcal)	Fat (g)	Saturated Fat (g)	Sodium (mg)	Carbs (g)	Fiber (g)	Protein (g)	Other
BREAKFAST Time:	**Portion**								
Breakfast Totals →									
SNACK Time:									
Snack Totals →									
LUNCH Time:									
Lunch Totals →									
SNACK Time:									
Snack Totals →									
DINNER Time:									
Dinner Totals →									
SNACK Time:									
Snack Totals →									
Daily Totals →									

DAILY FOOD GOALS

	target	actual	
			calories
			protein (g)
			carbs (g)
			fat (g)

water (8 oz glasses)

☐ ☐ ☐ ☐ ☐ ☐ ☐ ☐

fruits + vegetables (servings)

☐ ☐ ☐ ☐ ☐ ☐ ☐ ☐ ☐

FITNESS LOG

CARDIO/OTHER	Time of Day	Heart Rate	Duration	Speed	Level	Intensity	Other	Calories (kcal) Used
Calorie Totals								

WEIGHTS	Time of Day	Muscle Group	Reps	Sets	Duration	Intensity	Other	Calories (kcal) Used
Calorie Totals								
Total Calories Burned								

Calories Consumed - Calories Used = Net Calories - BMR (Basal Metabolic Rate) = Net Calorie Deficit

Vitamins/Supplements	Dosage	Quantity

mood
☹ 2 3 4 5 6 7 ☺

energy level
1 2 3 4 5 6 7 8

A 3,500 calorie deficit will equal 1 lb of weight loss.

Notes/Journal

FOOD LOG

Day	Date	Week #

		Calories (kcal)	Fat (g)	Saturated Fat (g)	Sodium (mg)	Carbs (g)	Fiber (g)	Protein (g)	Other
BREAKFAST Time:	Portion								
Breakfast Totals →									
SNACK Time:									
Snack Totals →									
LUNCH Time:									
Lunch Totals →									
SNACK Time:									
Snack Totals →									
DINNER Time:									
Dinner Totals →									
SNACK Time:									
Snack Totals →									
Daily Totals →									

DAILY FOOD GOALS

target	actual	
		calories
		protein (g)
		carbs (g)
		fat (g)

water (8 oz glasses)

☐ ☐ ☐ ☐ ☐ ☐ ☐ ☐

fruits + vegetables (servings)

☐ ☐ ☐ ☐ ☐ ☐ ☐ ☐ ☐

FITNESS LOG

CARDIO/OTHER	Time of Day	Heart Rate	Duration	Speed	Level	Intensity	Other	Calories (kcal) Used
Calorie Totals								

WEIGHTS	Time of Day	Muscle Group	Reps	Sets	Duration	Intensity	Other	Calories (kcal) Used
Calorie Totals								
Total Calories Burned								

Calories Consumed − Calories Used = Net Calories − BMR (Basal Metabolic Rate) = Net Calorie Deficit

Vitamins/Supplements	Dosage	Quantity

mood
☹ 2 3 4 5 6 7 ☺

energy level
1 2 3 4 5 6 7 8

A 3,500 calorie deficit will equal 1 lb of weight loss.

Notes/Journal

FOOD LOG

	Day	Date	Week #

	Portion	Calories (kcal)	Fat (g)	Saturated Fat (g)	Sodium (mg)	Carbs (g)	Fiber (g)	Protein (g)	Other
BREAKFAST Time:									
Breakfast Totals →									
SNACK Time:									
Snack Totals →									
LUNCH Time:									
Lunch Totals →									
SNACK Time:									
Snack Totals →									
DINNER Time:									
Dinner Totals →									
SNACK Time:									
Snack Totals →									
Daily Totals →									

DAILY FOOD GOALS

target	actual	
		calories
		protein (g)
		carbs (g)
		fat (g)

water (8 oz glasses)

☐ ☐ ☐ ☐ ☐ ☐ ☐ ☐

fruits + vegetables (servings)

☐ ☐ ☐ ☐ ☐ ☐ ☐ ☐ ☐

FITNESS LOG

CARDIO/OTHER	Time of Day	Heart Rate	Duration	Speed	Level	Intensity	Other	Calories (kcal) Used
Calorie Totals								

WEIGHTS	Time of Day	Muscle Group	Reps	Sets	Duration	Intensity	Other	Calories (kcal) Used
Calorie Totals								
Total Calories Burned								

Calories Consumed − Calories Used = Net Calories − BMR (Basal Metabolic Rate) = Net Calorie Deficit

Vitamins/Supplements	Dosage	Quantity

mood

☹ 2 3 4 5 6 7 ☺

energy level

1 2 3 4 5 6 7 8

A 3,500 calorie deficit will equal 1 lb of weight loss.

Notes/Journal

FOOD LOG

Day	Date	Week #

	Portion	Calories (kcal)	Fat (g)	Saturated Fat (g)	Sodium (mg)	Carbs (g)	Fiber (g)	Protein (g)	Other
BREAKFAST Time:									
Breakfast Totals →									
SNACK Time:									
Snack Totals →									
LUNCH Time:									
Lunch Totals →									
SNACK Time:									
Snack Totals →									
DINNER Time:									
Dinner Totals →									
SNACK Time:									
Snack Totals →									
Daily Totals →									

DAILY FOOD GOALS

target	actual	
		calories
		protein (g)
		carbs (g)
		fat (g)

water (8 oz glasses)

☐ ☐ ☐ ☐ ☐ ☐ ☐ ☐

fruits + vegetables (servings)

☐ ☐ ☐ ☐ ☐ ☐ ☐ ☐ ☐ ☐

FITNESS LOG

CARDIO/OTHER	Time of Day	Heart Rate	Duration	Speed	Level	Intensity	Other	Calories (kcal) Used
Calorie Totals								

WEIGHTS	Time of Day	Muscle Group	Reps	Sets	Duration	Intensity	Other	Calories (kcal) Used
Calorie Totals								

Total Calories Burned

Calories Consumed	−	Calories Used	=	Net Calories	−	BMR (Basal Metabolic Rate)	=	Net Calorie Deficit

Vitamins/Supplements	Dosage	Quantity

mood

☹ 2 3 4 5 6 7 ☺

energy level

1 2 3 4 5 6 7 8

A 3,500 calorie deficit will equal 1 lb of weight loss.

Notes/Journal

FOOD LOG

Day	Date	Week #

		Portion	Calories (kcal)	Fat (g)	Saturated Fat (g)	Sodium (mg)	Carbs (g)	Fiber (g)	Protein (g)	Other
BREAKFAST Time:										
Breakfast Totals →										
SNACK Time:										
Snack Totals →										
LUNCH Time:										
Lunch Totals →										
SNACK Time:										
Snack Totals →										
DINNER Time:										
Dinner Totals →										
SNACK Time:										
Snack Totals →										
Daily Totals →										

DAILY FOOD GOALS

	target	actual	
			calories
			protein (g)
			carbs (g)
			fat (g)

water (8 oz glasses)

☐ ☐ ☐ ☐ ☐ ☐ ☐ ☐

fruits + vegetables (servings)

☐ ☐ ☐ ☐ ☐ ☐ ☐ ☐ ☐

FITNESS LOG

CARDIO/OTHER	Time of Day	Heart Rate	Duration	Speed	Level	Intensity	Other	Calories (kcal) Used
Calorie Totals								

WEIGHTS	Time of Day	Muscle Group	Reps	Sets	Duration	Intensity	Other	Calories (kcal) Used
Calorie Totals								
Total Calories Burned								

Calories Consumed - Calories Used = Net Calories - BMR (Basal Metabolic Rate) = Net Calorie Deficit

Vitamins/Supplements	Dosage	Quantity

mood
☹ 2 3 4 5 6 7 ☺

energy level
1 2 3 4 5 6 7 8

A 3,500 calorie deficit will equal 1 lb of weight loss.

Notes/Journal

FOOD LOG

Day	Date	Week #

		Calories (kcal)	Fat (g)	Saturated Fat (g)	Sodium (mg)	Carbs (g)	Fiber (g)	Protein (g)	Other
BREAKFAST Time:	Portion								
Breakfast Totals →									
SNACK Time:									
Snack Totals →									
LUNCH Time:									
Lunch Totals →									
SNACK Time:									
Snack Totals →									
DINNER Time:									
Dinner Totals →									
SNACK Time:									
Snack Totals →									
Daily Totals →									

DAILY FOOD GOALS

target	actual	
		calories
		protein (g)
		carbs (g)
		fat (g)

water (8 oz glasses)

☐☐☐☐☐☐☐☐☐

fruits + vegetables (servings)

☐☐☐☐☐☐☐☐☐☐

FITNESS LOG

CARDIO/OTHER	Time of Day	Heart Rate	Duration	Speed	Level	Intensity	Other	Calories (kcal) Used
Calorie Totals								

WEIGHTS	Time of Day	Muscle Group	Reps	Sets	Duration	Intensity	Other	Calories (kcal) Used
Calorie Totals								

Total Calories Burned

Calories Consumed	-	Calories Used	=	Net Calories	-	BMR (Basal Metabolic Rate)	=	Net Calorie Deficit

Vitamins/Supplements	Dosage	Quantity

mood

☹ 2 3 4 5 6 7 ☺

energy level

1 2 3 4 5 6 7 8

A 3,500 calorie deficit will equal 1 lb of weight loss.

Notes/Journal

WEEKLY PROGRESS

	Weight	BMI	BMR	Heart Rate	Cholesterol	Blood Sugar	Other
STATS							
Last Week							
Current							

	Neck	Shoulder	Chest	Waist	Hip	Thigh	Calf	Arm	Other
MEASUREMENTS									
Last Week									
Current									

Notes/Journal

_____
_____
_____
_____
_____
_____
_____
_____
_____
_____
_____

GOALS FOR NEXT WEEK

_____
_____
_____
_____
_____
_____
_____
_____
_____
_____

DAILY CALORIE DEFICIT

Day 1		Day 5	
Day 2		Day 6	
Day 3		Day 7	
Day 4		Weekly Total	

Waist Hip Ratio

Women <.7
Men   <.9

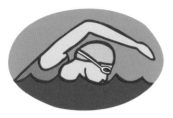

Physical fitness is not only one of the most important keys to a healthy body, it is the basis of dynamic and creative intellectual activity.

JOHN F. KENNEDY

TIP OF THE WEEK

Both strengh-training *and* cardio are essential for dropping pounds and keeping them off, though. I think of aerobic exercise as the kindling in a fire and resistance exercise as the big logs that keep it burning. Cardio melts calories on the spot, while toning gives you stronger muscles that burn more calories all day long, so it's easier to slim down for good.

—Bob Greene

FOOD LOG

Day	Date	Week #

	Portion	Calories (kcal)	Fat (g)	Saturated Fat (g)	Sodium (mg)	Carbs (g)	Fiber (g)	Protein (g)	Other
BREAKFAST Time:									
Breakfast Totals →									
SNACK Time:									
Snack Totals →									
LUNCH Time:									
Lunch Totals →									
SNACK Time:									
Snack Totals →									
DINNER Time:									
Dinner Totals →									
SNACK Time:									
Snack Totals →									
Daily Totals →									

DAILY FOOD GOALS

target	actual	
		calories
		protein (g)
		carbs (g)
		fat (g)

water (8 oz glasses)

☐ ☐ ☐ ☐ ☐ ☐ ☐ ☐

fruits + vegetables (servings)

☐ ☐ ☐ ☐ ☐ ☐ ☐ ☐ ☐ ☐

FITNESS LOG

CARDIO/OTHER	Time of Day	Heart Rate	Duration	Speed	Level	Intensity	Other	Calories (kcal) Used
.								
Calorie Totals								

WEIGHTS	Time of Day	Muscle Group	Reps	Sets	Duration	Intensity	Other	Calories (kcal) Used
Calorie Totals								
Total Calories Burned								

Calories Consumed	−	Calories Used	=	Net Calories	−	BMR (Basal Metabolic Rate)	=	Net Calorie Deficit

Vitamins/Supplements	Dosage	Quantity

mood

☹ 2 3 4 5 6 7 ☺

energy level

1 2 3 4 5 6 7 8

A 3,500 calorie deficit will equal 1 lb of weight loss.

Notes/Journal

FOOD LOG

	Day		Date		Week #

		Calories (kcal)	Fat (g)	Saturated Fat (g)	Sodium (mg)	Carbs (g)	Fiber (g)	Protein (g)	Other
BREAKFAST Time:	Portion								
Breakfast Totals →									
SNACK Time:									
Snack Totals →									
LUNCH Time:									
Lunch Totals →									
SNACK Time:									
Snack Totals →									
DINNER Time:									
Dinner Totals →									
SNACK Time:									
Snack Totals →									
Daily Totals →									

DAILY FOOD GOALS

target	actual	
		calories
		protein (g)
		carbs (g)
		fat (g)

water (8 oz glasses)

☐☐☐☐☐☐☐☐

fruits + vegetables (servings)

☐☐☐☐☐☐☐☐☐

FITNESS LOG

CARDIO/OTHER	Time of Day	Heart Rate	Duration	Speed	Level	Intensity	Other	Calories (kcal) Used
Calorie Totals								

WEIGHTS	Time of Day	Muscle Group	Reps	Sets	Duration	Intensity	Other	Calories (kcal) Used
Calorie Totals								

Total Calories Burned

Calories Consumed	−	Calories Used	=	Net Calories	−	BMR (Basal Metabolic Rate)	=	Net Calorie Deficit

Vitamins/Supplements	Dosage	Quantity

mood

☹ 2 3 4 5 6 7 ☺

energy level

1 2 3 4 5 6 7 8

A 3,500 calorie deficit will equal 1 lb of weight loss.

Notes/Journal

FOOD LOG

Day	Date	Week #

		Calories (kcal)	Fat (g)	Saturated Fat (g)	Sodium (mg)	Carbs (g)	Fiber (g)	Protein (g)	Other
BREAKFAST Time:	Portion								
Breakfast Totals →									
SNACK Time:									
Snack Totals →									
LUNCH Time:									
Lunch Totals →									
SNACK Time:									
Snack Totals →									
DINNER Time:									
Dinner Totals →									
SNACK Time:									
Snack Totals →									
Daily Totals →									

DAILY FOOD GOALS

target	actual	
		calories
		protein (g)
		carbs (g)
		fat (g)

water (8 oz glasses)

☐☐☐☐☐☐☐☐

fruits + vegetables (servings)

☐☐☐☐☐☐☐☐☐

FITNESS LOG

CARDIO/OTHER	Time of Day	Heart Rate	Duration	Speed	Level	Intensity	Other	Calories (kcal) Used
Calorie Totals								

WEIGHTS	Time of Day	Muscle Group	Reps	Sets	Duration	Intensity	Other	Calories (kcal) Used
Calorie Totals								

Total Calories Burned

Calories Consumed	-	Calories Used	=	Net Calories	-	BMR (Basal Metabolic Rate)	=	Net Calorie Deficit

Vitamins/Supplements	Dosage	Quantity

mood

☹ 2 3 4 5 6 7 ☺

energy level

1 2 3 4 5 6 7 8

A 3,500 calorie deficit will equal 1 lb of weight loss.

Notes/Journal

FOOD LOG

Day	Date	Week #

	Portion	Calories (kcal)	Fat (g)	Saturated Fat (g)	Sodium (mg)	Carbs (g)	Fiber (g)	Protein (g)	Other
BREAKFAST Time:									
Breakfast Totals →									
SNACK Time:									
Snack Totals →									
LUNCH Time:									
Lunch Totals →									
SNACK Time:									
Snack Totals →									
DINNER Time:									
Dinner Totals →									
SNACK Time:									
Snack Totals →									
Daily Totals →									

DAILY FOOD GOALS

	target	actual
calories		
protein (g)		
carbs (g)		
fat (g)		

water (8 oz glasses)

☐ ☐ ☐ ☐ ☐ ☐ ☐ ☐

fruits + vegetables (servings)

☐ ☐ ☐ ☐ ☐ ☐ ☐ ☐ ☐ ☐

FITNESS LOG

CARDIO/OTHER	Time of Day	Heart Rate	Duration	Speed	Level	Intensity	Other	Calories (kcal) Used
Calorie Totals								

WEIGHTS	Time of Day	Muscle Group	Reps	Sets	Duration	Intensity	Other	Calories (kcal) Used
Calorie Totals								

Total Calories Burned

Calories Consumed	−	Calories Used	=	Net Calories	−	BMR (Basal Metabolic Rate)	=	Net Calorie Deficit

Vitamins/Supplements	Dosage	Quantity

mood

☹ 2 3 4 5 6 7 ☺

energy level

1 2 3 4 5 6 7 8

A 3,500 calorie deficit will equal 1 lb of weight loss.

Notes/Journal

FOOD LOG

Day	Date	Week #

	Calories (kcal)	Fat (g)	Saturated Fat (g)	Sodium (mg)	Carbs (g)	Fiber (g)	Protein (g)	Other
BREAKFAST Time: Portion								
Breakfast Totals →								
SNACK Time:								
Snack Totals →								
LUNCH Time:								
Lunch Totals →								
SNACK Time:								
Snack Totals →								
DINNER Time:								
Dinner Totals →								
SNACK Time:								
Snack Totals →								
Daily Totals →								

DAILY FOOD GOALS

target	actual	
		calories
		protein (g)
		carbs (g)
		fat (g)

water (8 oz glasses)

☐ ☐ ☐ ☐ ☐ ☐ ☐ ☐

fruits + vegetables (servings)

☐ ☐ ☐ ☐ ☐ ☐ ☐ ☐ ☐

FITNESS LOG

CARDIO/OTHER	Time of Day	Heart Rate	Duration	Speed	Level	Intensity	Other	Calories (kcal) Used
Calorie Totals								

WEIGHTS	Time of Day	Muscle Group	Reps	Sets	Duration	Intensity	Other	Calories (kcal) Used
Calorie Totals								
Total Calories Burned								

Calories Consumed – Calories Used = Net Calories – BMR (Basal Metabolic Rate) = Net Calorie Deficit

Vitamins/Supplements	Dosage	Quantity

mood

☹ 2 3 4 5 6 7 ☺

energy level

1 2 3 4 5 6 7 8

A 3,500 calorie deficit will equal 1 lb of weight loss.

Notes/Journal

FOOD LOG

	Day		Date		Week #

			Calories (kcal)	Fat (g)	Saturated Fat (g)	Sodium (mg)	Carbs (g)	Fiber (g)	Protein (g)	Other
BREAKFAST Time:		Portion								
Breakfast Totals	→									
SNACK Time:										
Snack Totals	→									
LUNCH Time:										
Lunch Totals	→									
SNACK Time:										
Snack Totals	→									
DINNER Time:										
Dinner Totals	→									
SNACK Time:										
Snack Totals	→									
Daily Totals	→									

DAILY FOOD GOALS

target	actual	
		calories
		protein (g)
		carbs (g)
		fat (g)

water (8 oz glasses)

☐ ☐ ☐ ☐ ☐ ☐ ☐ ☐ ☐ ☐

fruits + vegetables (servings)

☐ ☐ ☐ ☐ ☐ ☐ ☐ ☐ ☐ ☐

FITNESS LOG

CARDIO/OTHER	Time of Day	Heart Rate	Duration	Speed	Level	Intensity	Other	Calories (kcal) Used
Calorie Totals								

WEIGHTS	Time of Day	Muscle Group	Reps	Sets	Duration	Intensity	Other	Calories (kcal) Used
Calorie Totals								
Total Calories Burned								

Calories Consumed		Calories Used		Net Calories		BMR (Basal Metabolic Rate)		Net Calorie Deficit
	−		=		−		=	

Vitamins/Supplements	Dosage	Quantity

mood
☹ 2 3 4 5 6 7 ☺

energy level
1 2 3 4 5 6 7 8

A 3,500 calorie deficit will equal 1 lb of weight loss.

Notes/Journal

FOOD LOG

Day	Date	Week #

	Portion	Calories (kcal)	Fat (g)	Saturated Fat (g)	Sodium (mg)	Carbs (g)	Fiber (g)	Protein (g)	Other
BREAKFAST Time:									
Breakfast Totals →									
SNACK Time:									
Snack Totals →									
LUNCH Time:									
Lunch Totals →									
SNACK Time:									
Snack Totals →									
DINNER Time:									
Dinner Totals →									
SNACK Time:									
Snack Totals →									
Daily Totals →									

DAILY FOOD GOALS

target	actual	
		calories
		protein (g)
		carbs (g)
		fat (g)

water (8 oz glasses)

☐ ☐ ☐ ☐ ☐ ☐ ☐ ☐

fruits + vegetables (servings)

☐ ☐ ☐ ☐ ☐ ☐ ☐ ☐ ☐ ☐

FITNESS LOG

CARDIO/OTHER	Time of Day	Heart Rate	Duration	Speed	Level	Intensity	Other	Calories (kcal) Used
Calorie Totals								

WEIGHTS	Time of Day	Muscle Group	Reps	Sets	Duration	Intensity	Other	Calories (kcal) Used
Calorie Totals								
Total Calories Burned								

Calories Consumed − Calories Used = Net Calories − BMR (Basal Metabolic Rate) = Net Calorie Deficit

Vitamins/Supplements	Dosage	Quantity

mood
☹ 2 3 4 5 6 7 ☺

energy level
1 2 3 4 5 6 7 8

A 3,500 calorie deficit will equal 1 lb of weight loss.

Notes/Journal

WEEKLY PROGRESS

	Weight	BMI	BMR	Heart Rate	Cholesterol	Blood Sugar	Other
STATS							
Last Week							
Current							

	Neck	Shoulder	Chest	Waist	Hip	Thigh	Calf	Arm	Other
MEASUREMENTS									
Last Week									
Current									

Notes/Journal

GOALS FOR NEXT WEEK

DAILY CALORIE DEFICIT

Day 1		Day 5	
Day 2		Day 6	
Day 3		Day 7	
Day 4		Weekly Total	

Waist Hip Ratio

Women <.7
Men   <.9

NUTRITIONAL facts for POPULAR FOODS

One should eat to live,
and not live to eat.

MOLIÈRE

Description of food	Calories	Fat	Saturated Fat
	(kcal)	(Grams)	(Grams)
ACORN SQUASH, fresh, cubed, 1 cup/150g	56	0	0
ALMONDS, raw, 10	69	6	0
ANCHOVY, European, fresh, 3 oz/85g	111	4	1
APPLE, fresh, whole, 1 med	95	0	0
APPLE JUICE, canned or bottled (unsweetened), 8 fl oz/240mL	114	0	0
APPLESAUCE, sweetened, w/o salt, 1 cup/246g	167	0	0
APPLESAUCE, unsweetened, 1 cup/244g	102	0	0
APRICOTS, dried, uncooked, halves, 1 cup/130g	313	1	0
APRICOTS, fresh, whole, 1 med	17	0	0
ARTICHOKES, fresh, whole, 1 med	60	0	0
ASPARAGUS, fresh, cut, 1/2 cup/67g	13	0	0
AVOCADO, California, fresh, whole, 1 fruit	227	21	3
BACON, Canadian style, grilled, 1 oz (28g) slice	43	2	1
BACON, pan fried, 1 slice	42	3	1
BAGEL, plain (3"/8cm diameter), 1 bagel	146	1	0
BAKED BEANS, homemade, 1 cup/253g	392	13	5
BAKED BEANS, vegetarian, 1 cup/254g	239	1	0
BANANA, whole, 1 med	105	0	0
BARLEY, pearled, cooked, 1 cup/157g	193	1	0
BEEF, brisket, point half, 1/8"/.3cm fat, all grades, braised, 3 oz/85g	297	23	9
BEEF, ground, 25% fat, patty, broiled, 3 oz/85g	236	16	6
BEEF, rib eye, small end, 0" fat, all grades, broiled, 1 steak	576	34	13
BEEF, top sirloin, 1/8"/.3cm fat, all grades, broiled, 3 oz /85g	207	12	5
BEEF BROTH, canned, 1 cup/240mL	17	1	0
BEEF STEW, canned, 1 serving	220	12	5
BEER, light, all, 12 fl oz/355mL	103	0	0
BEER, regular, all, 12 fl oz/355mL	153	0	0
BEETS, fresh (2"/5cm diameter), 1 beet	35	0	0
BISCUITS, plain or buttermilk, commercial (2.5"/6.4cm diameter), 1 biscuit	128	6	1
BLACK BEANS, boiled, 1 cup/172g	227	1	0
BLACKBERRIES, fresh, 1 cup/144g	62	1	0
BOLOGNA, beef, 1 oz (28g) slice	87	8	3
BOYSENBERRIES, frozen, unsweetened, 1 cup/132g	66	0	0

Sodium	Carbs	Fiber	Protein
(Milligrams)	(Grams)	(Grams)	(Grams)
4	15	2	1
0	3	2	3
88	0	0	17
1	25	4	0
10	28	0	0
5	43	3	0
5	28	3	0
13	81	9	4
0	4	1	0
120	13	7	4
1	3	1	1
11	12	9	3
363	0	0	6
188	0	0	3
255	29	1	6
1068	55	14	14
871	54	10	12
1	27	3	1
5	44	6	4
59	0	0	21
66	0	0	22
130	0	0	64
48	0	0	23
782	0	0	3
947	16	4	11
14	6	0	1
14	13	0	2
64	8	2	1
368	17	0	2
2	41	15	15
1	14	8	2
302	1	0	3
1	16	7	1

Description of food	Calories	Fat	Saturated Fat
	(kcal)	(Grams)	(Grams)
BREAD, French or Vienna, 2"/5cm slice	92	1	0
BREAD, Italian, 1 slice	54	1	0
BREAD, multi-grain, 1 slice	69	1	0
BREAD, rye, 1 slice	83	1	0
BREAD, wheat, 1 slice	66	1	0
BREAD, white, commercial, 1 slice	66	1	0
BREAD STUFFING, dry mix, prepared, 1 oz/28g	50	2	0
BROCCOLI, boiled, chopped, 1/2 cup/78g	27	0	0
BROCCOLI, fresh, chopped, 1 cup/88g	31	0	0
BROWNIES, commercial (2-3/4"/7cm sq), 1	227	9	2
BRUSSELS SPROUTS, boiled, 1/2 cup/78g	28	0	0
BUTTER, salted, 1 tbsp/14g	102	12	7
BUTTERNUT SQUASH, baked, cubed, 1 cup/205g	82	0	0
BUTTERNUT SQUASH, frozen, boiled, mashed, 1 cup/240g	94	0	0
CABBAGE, common, fresh, shredded, 1 cup/70g	17	0	0
CABBAGE, red, fresh, shredded, 1 cup/70g	22	0	0
CAKE, angel food, commercial (12 oz/340g cake), 1/12 cake	72	0	0
CAKE, cheesecake, commercial (17 oz/482g cake),1/6 cake	257	18	8
CAKE, chocolate, commercial, w/ chocolate frosting (18 oz/510g cake), 1/8 cake	235	10	3
CAKE, yellow, commercial, w/ vanilla frosting (18 oz/510g cake), 1/8 cake	239	9	2
CANDY, caramels, 1 pc	39	1	0
CANTALOUPE, fresh, cubed, 1 cup/160g	54	0	0
CARROT, baby, fresh, 1 med	4	0	0
CARROT, fresh, whole, 1 med	25	0	0
CASHEW NUTS, dry roasted, w/ salt, halves, 1 cup/137g	786	64	13
CATSUP, 1 tbsp/15g	15	0	0
CAULIFLOWER, boiled (1"/3cm pcs), 1/2 cup/62g	14	0	0
CAULIFLOWER, fresh, 1 cup/107g	25	0	0
CELERY, fresh, chopped, 1 cup/101g	16	0	0
CHEESE, American, pasteurized, processed, 3/4 oz/21g slice	79	7	4
CHEESE, blue, 1 oz/28g	100	8	5
CHEESE, cheddar, 1 oz/28g slice	113	9	6

Sodium	Carbs	Fiber	Protein
(Milligrams)	(Grams)	(Grams)	(Grams)
208	18	1	4
117	10	1	2
109	11	2	3
211	15	2	3
130	12	1	3
170	13	1	2
154	6	1	1
32	6	3	2
30	6	2	3
175	36	1	3
16	6	2	2
91	0	0	0
8	22	0	2
5	24	0	3
13	4	2	1
19	5	1	1
210	16	0	2
166	20	0	4
214	35	2	3
220	38	0	2
25	8	0	0
26	13	1	1
8	1	0	0
42	6	2	1
877	45	4	21
167	4	0	0
9	3	1	1
30	5	3	2
81	3	2	1
313	0	0	5
395	1	0	6
174	0	0	7

Description of food	Calories	Fat	Saturated Fat
	(kcal)	(Grams)	(Grams)
CHEESE, cottage creamed, small curd, 1/2 cup/113g	110	5	2
CHEESE, cream, 1 tbsp/15g	50	5	3
CHEESE, feta, 1 oz/28g	75	6	4
CHEESE, goat, soft, 1 oz/28g	76	6	4
CHEESE, Mozzarella, part skim milk, 1oz/28g	72	5	3
CHEESE, Muenster, 1 oz/28g slice	103	8	5
CHEESE, Parmesan, grated, 1 tbsp/5g	22	1	1
CHEESE, ricotta, part skim milk, 1 oz/28g	39	2	1
CHEESE, Swiss, 1 oz/28g slice	106	8	5
CHERRIES, sweet, fresh, 1 cup/138g	87	0	0
CHICKEN BREAST, fat free mesquite flavored, slices, 2 slices	34	0	0
CHICKEN, broiler/fryer, back, meat only, roasted, 1 back	191	11	3
CHICKEN, broiler/fryer, drumstick, meat only, fried	82	3	1
CHICKPEAS, boiled, 1 cup/164g	269	4	0
CHOCOLATE MILK, commercial, 1 cup/240mL	208	8	5
CLAMS, breaded & fried, 3 oz/85g	172	9	2
CLEMENTINES, fresh, whole, 1 fruit	35	0	0
COFFEE, brewed, 1 cup/240mL	2	0	0
COOKIES, chocolate chip, commercial, lower fat, 1	45	2	0
COOKIES, graham crackers, plain, honey, or cinnamon (2.5"/6cm sq), 1	30	1	0
COOKIES, oatmeal, commercial (3.5"/9cm diameter), 1	112	5	1
COOKIES, peanut butter, commercial, 1	72	4	1
COOKIES, shortbread, plain, commercial (1-5/8"/4cm sq), 1	40	2	0
CORN, yellow, boiled, w/o salt, 1 cup/149g	143	2	0
CORNBREAD, homemade, made w/ 2% milk, 1 pc	173	5	1
CRAB, Alaska King, cooked in moist heat, 3 oz/85g	82	1	0
CRACKERS, matzo, plain, 1 matzo	111	0	0
CRACKERS, oyster, 5 crackers	21	0	0
CRACKERS, saltine, 5 crackers	63	1	0
CRANBERRIES, fresh, 1 cup/100g	46	0	0
CRANBERRY SAUCE, canned, sweetened, 1 cup/277g	418	0	0
CUCUMBER, peeled, fresh, slices, 1 cup/119g	14	0	0

Sodium	Carbs	Fiber	Protein
(Milligrams)	(Grams)	(Grams)	(Grams)
410	4	0	13
47	1	0	1
316	1	0	4
104	0	0	5
175	1	0	7
176	0	0	7
76	0	0	2
35	1	0	3
54	2	0	8
0	22	3	1
437	1	0	7
77	0	0	23
40	0	0	12
11	45	13	15
150	26	2	8
309	9	0	12
1	9	1	1
5	0	0	0
38	7	0	1
42	5	0	0
96	17	1	2
62	9	0	1
36	5	0	0
0	31	4	5
428	28	0	4
911	0	0	16
1	23	1	3
56	4	0	0
167	11	0	1
2	12	5	0
80	108	3	1
2	3	1	1

Description of food	Calories	Fat	Saturated Fat
	(kcal)	(Grams)	(Grams)
CUPCAKE, chocolate, w/ frosting, 1 cupcake	131	2	0
DANISH PASTRY, almond (4.25"/ 11cm diameter), 1 pastry	280	16	4
DANISH PASTRY, cheese, 1 pastry	266	16	5
DOUGHNUT, cake type, plain (3.25"/8cm diameter), 1	226	13	4
DOUGHNUT HOLE, glazed, 1	52	2	1
DOUGHNUT, old fashioned, plain (3.25 "/8cm diameter), 1	226	13	4
DUCK, w/ skin, roasted, chopped, 1 cup/140g	472	40	14
ECLAIR, custard filled, w/ chocolate glaze, home-made, 1	262	16	4
EDAMAME, frozen, 1 cup/155g	189	8	1
EGGPLANT, fresh, cubed, 1 cup/82g	20	0	0
EGG WHITE, 1/4 cup/61g	30	0	0
EGGS, fried, 1 lg	90	7	2
EGGS, hard-boiled, 1 lg	78	5	2
EGGS, scrambled, 1 lg	102	7	2
ENGLISH MUFFIN, plain, toasted, 1	140	1	0
FAVA BEANS, boiled, 1 cup/170g	187	1	0
FIG, fresh, whole, 1 lg	47	0	0
FISH STICKS, frozen, preheated, 1 stick	70	4	1
FRANKFURTER, beef (5"/13cm long x 3/4"/2cm diameter), 1	148	13	5
FRANKFURTER, chicken, 1	100	7	2
FRENCH TOAST, homemade, w/ 2% milk, 1 slice	149	7	2
FRUIT SALAD, canned, in heavy syrup, 1 cup/255g	186	0	0
FRUIT SALAD, canned, in water, 1 cup/245g	74	0	0
GARBANZO BEANS, boiled, 1 cup/164g	269	4	0
GRAPE JUICE, canned or bottled, 8 fl oz/240mL	152	0	0
GRAPEFRUIT, pink & red, Florida, fresh, 1/2 fruit	37	0	0
GRAPES, American type, 1 cup/92g	62	0	0
GREEN BEANS, fresh, cooked w/o salt, 1 cup/125g	44	0	0
GUAVA, fresh, 1 fruit	37	1	0

Sodium	Carbs	Fiber	Protein
(Milligrams)	(Grams)	(Grams)	(Grams)
178	29	2	2
236	30	1	5
320	26	1	6
301	25	1	3
50	7	0	1
301	25	1	3
83	0	0	27
337	24	1	6
9	15	8	17
2	5	3	1
101	0	0	6
94	0	0	6
62	1	0	6
171	1	0	7
248	27	2	5
8	33	9	13
1	12	2	0
118	6	0	3
513	2	0	5
380	1	0	7
311	16	0	5
15	49	3	1
7	19	3	1
11	45	13	15
13	37	0	1
0	9	1	1
2	16	1	1
1	10	4	2
1	8	3	1

Description of food	Calories	Fat	Saturated Fat
	(kcal)	(Grams)	(Grams)
HAM, boneless, reg (approx 11% fat), roasted, 3 oz/85g	151	8	3
HAM, chopped, from fresh, 1 oz/28g	50	3	1
HAM, whole, lean & fat, roasted, 3 oz/85g	207	14	5
HONEY, 1 tbsp/21g	64	0	0
HONEYDEW, fresh, diced, 1 cup/170g	61	0	0
HUMMUS, commercial, 1 tbsp/15g	25	1	0
ICE CREAM, chocolate, 1/2 cup/66g	143	7	4
ICE CREAM, vanilla, 1/2 cup/66g	137	7.2	4
JAMS & PRESERVES, other than apricot, 1 tbsp/20g	56	0	0
JELLIES, 1 tbsp/21g	56	0	0
JICAMA, fresh, slices, 1 cup/120g	46	0	0
KALE, fresh, chopped, 1 cup/67g	34	0	0
KIDNEY BEANS, California red, boiled, 1 cup/177g	219	0	0
KIWI FRUIT, fresh, w/o skin, 1 fruit	56	0	0
KOHLRABI, fresh, 1 cup/135g	36	0	0
LAMB, Australian, leg, shank half, 1/8"/.3cm fat, roasted, 3 oz/85g	196	12	5
LAMB, ground, broiled, 3 oz/85g	241	17	7
LASAGNA, vegetable, frozen, baked, 1 cup/226g	314	14	5
LEEK, fresh, 1 leek	54	0	0
LENTILS, boiled, 1 cup/198g	230	1	0
LETTUCE, romaine, shredded, 1 cup/47g	8	0	0
LIMA BEANS, fresh, baby, 1/2 cup/101g	88	1	0
LOBSTER, northern, cooked in moist heat, 3 oz/85g	83	1	0
LOGANBERRIES, frozen, 1 cup/147g	81	0	0
MACKEREL, Atlantic, cooked in dry heat, 3 oz/85g	223	15	4
MANGO, fresh, 1 fruit	135	1	0
MAPLE SYRUP, 1 tbsp/20g	52	0	0
MARGARINE, 80% fat, composite, stick, w/ salt, 1 tbsp/15g	100	11	2
MARSHMALLOW, 1 reg	23	0	0
MAYONNAISE, cholesterol free, 1 tbsp/14g	103	12	2

Sodium	Carbs	Fiber	Protein
(Milligrams)	(Grams)	(Grams)	(Grams)
1275	0	0	19
372	1	0	5
1009	0	0	18
1	17	0	0
31	15	1	1
57	2	1	1
50	19	1	3
53	16	0.5	2
6	14	0	0
6	15	0	0
5	11	6	1
29	7	1	2
7	40	17	16
3	13	3	1
27	8	5	2
57	0	0	21
69	0	0	21
796	32	4	16
18	13	2	1
4	40	16	18
4	2	1	1
6	16	4	5
323	1	0	17
1	19	8	2
71	0	0	20
4	35	4	1
2	13	0	0
132	0	0	0
6	6	0	0
73	0	0	0

Description of food	Calories	Fat	Saturated Fat
	(kcal)	(Grams)	(Grams)
MAYONNAISE, light, 1 tbsp/15g	49	5	1
MILK, low fat, 1% milkfat, 1 cup/240mL	102	2	2
MILK, reduced fat, 2% milkfat, 1 cup/240mL	122	5	3
MILK, skim, 1 cup/240mL	83	0	0
MILK SHAKE, thick, chocolate, 8 fl oz/240mL	270	6	4
MILLET, cooked, 1 cup/174g	207	2	0
MIXED VEGETABLES, canned, drained, 1 cup/163g	80	0	0
MOLASSES, 1 tbsp/20g	58	0	0
MUFFIN, blueberry, commercial (2.75"/7cm diameter), 1	259	13	2
MUFFIN, corn, commercial, small, 1	201	6	1
MUSHROOMS, canned, 1 cup/156g	39	0	0
MUSHROOMS, portabella, grilled, slices, 1 cup/121g	42	1	0
MUSHROOMS, white, fresh pcs, 1 cup/70g	15	0	0
NAVY BEANS, boiled, 1 cup/182g	255	1	0
NECTARINE, fresh, whole, 1 sm	57	0	0
NOODLES, egg, 1 cup/160g	221	3	1
OLIVE OIL, salad or cooking, 1 tbsp/14g	119	14	2
OLIVES, pickled, canned or bottled, 1 olive	4	0	0
ONION, sweet, fresh, 1 onion	106	0	0
ONIONS, fresh, chopped, 1 cup/160g	64	0	0
ORANGE, fresh, all varieties (2-5/8"/7cm diameter), 1 fruit	62	0	0
ORANGE JUICE, fresh, 1 cup/240mL	112	1	0
PANCAKE, plain, homemade (4"/10cm diameter), 1	86	4	1
PAPAYA, fresh, cubed, 1 cup/140g	55	0	0
PARSNIPS, boiled, slices, 1 cup/156g	111	0	0
PASTA, spaghetti, cooked, 1 cup/140g	221	1	0
PASTA, spaghetti, whole wheat, cooked, 1 cup/140g	174	1	0
PEACH, fresh (2-1/2"/6cm diameter), 1 fruit	51	0	0
PEACHES, canned in juice, 1 cup/250g	110	0	0
PEANUT BUTTER, chunky, w/ salt, 2 tbsp/32g	188	16	3
PEANUT BUTTER, smooth, w/ salt, 2 tbsp/32g	188	16	3
PEAR, fresh, whole, 1 sm	86	0	0
PEAS, boiled, 1/2 cup/80g	34	0	0

Sodium	Carbs	Fiber	Protein
(Milligrams)	(Grams)	(Grams)	(Grams)
106	1	0	0
107	12	0	8
100	11	0	8
115	12	0	8
102	48	1	7
3	41	2	6
243	15	5	4
7	15	0	0
208	33	1	3
344	34	2	4
663	8	4	3
12	6	3	5
4	2	1	2
0	47	19	15
0	14	2	1
8	40	2	7
0	0	0	0
40	0	0	0
26	25	3	3
6	15	3	2
0	15	3	1
2	26	1	2
167	11	0	2
4	14	3	1
16	27	6	2
1	43	3	8
4	37	6	7
0	12	2	1
10	29	3	2
156	7	3	8
147	6	2	8
1	23	5	1
3	6	2	3

Description of food	Calories	Fat	Saturated Fat
	(kcal)	(Grams)	(Grams)
PEAS, green, fresh, 1/2 cup/72g	59	0	0
PEPPERONI, pork, beef, 1 oz/28g	138	12	4
PEPPER, sweet, yellow, fresh, 1 lg	50	0	0
PEPPERS, sweet, green, fresh, chopped, 1 cup/149g	30	0	0
PERSIMMON, native, fresh, 1 fruit	32	0	0
PICKLE, cucumber, sour (4"/10cm long), 1 pickle	15	0	0
PICKLE, cucumber, sweet, gherkin (3"/8cm long), 1 pickle	32	0	0
PICKLE RELISH, hamburger, 1 tbsp/15g	19	0	0
PIE, apple, homemade (9"/23cm diameter), 1/8 pie	411	19	5
PIE, blueberry, commercial (9"/23cm diameter), 1/8 pie	290	13	2
PINEAPPLE, fresh, traditional varieties, chunks, 1 cup/165g	74	0	0
PINTO BEANS, boiled, 1 cup/171g	245	1	0
PITA BREAD, white (6-1/2"/7cm diameter), 1 pita	165	1	0
PIZZA, cheese, 1 slice (3.6 oz/119g)	317	12	5
PLUM, fresh (2-1/8"/5cm diameter), 1 fruit	30	0	0
PLUMS, canned in juice, 1 cup/252g	146	0	0
POPCORN, air popped, 1oz/28g	108	1	0
POPCORN, oil popped, 1oz/28g	146	8	1
PORK, ground, cooked, 3 oz/85g	252	18	7
PORK LOIN, blade chops, broiled, 3 oz/85g	272	21	8
PORK SPARERIBS, roasted, 3 oz/85g	303	26	8
POTATO CHIPS, bbq, 1 oz/28g	139	9	2
POTATO CHIPS, plain, made from dried potatoes, reduced fat, 1 oz/28g	141	18	1
POTATOES, french fried, frozen, oven heated, w/o salt, 10 fries	166	9	3
POTATOES, hashed browns, homemade, 1 cup/156g	413	20	3
POTATOES, mashed, homemade, whole milk added, 1 cup/210g	174	1	1
PRETZELS, hard, plain, salted, 1 oz/28g	108	1	0
PRUNES, dehydrated, stewed, 1 cup/280g	316	1	0
PRUNES, uncooked, 1 cup/174g	418	1	0
PUDDING, chocolate, reg, prepared w/ whole milk, 1/2 cup/142g	169	4	3
PUDDING, vanilla, ready to eat, 4oz/110g	143	4	1
PUMPKIN, boiled, mashed, 1 cup/245g	49	0	0
PUMPKIN SEEDS, dried, 1 oz/28g	151	13	2

Sodium	Carbs	Fiber	Protein
(Milligrams)	(Grams)	(Grams)	(Grams)
4	10	4	4
463	0	0	6
4	12	2	2
4	7	3	1
0	8	0	0
1631	3	2	0
160	7	0	0
164	5	1	0
327	58	0	4
406	44	1	2
2	19	0	1
2	45	15	15
322	33	1	5
712	39	2	14
0	8	1	0
3	38	2	1
2	22	4	4
1	16	3	3
62	0	0	22
60	0	0	19
77	0	0	18
213	15	1	2
115	18	1	1
307	20	2	2
534	55	5	5
634	37	3	4
380	22	1	3
6	83	0	3
3	111	12	4
136	28	1	5
156	25	0	2
2	12	3	2
5	5	1	7

Description of food	Calories	Fat	Saturated Fat
	(kcal)	(Grams)	(Grams)
QUINOA, cooked, 1 cup/185g	222	4	0
RADISHES, fresh, slices, 1 cup/116g	19	0	0
RAISINS, purple, seedless, 1 cup/165g	493	1	0
RASPBERRIES, fresh, 1 cup/123g	64	1	0
RICE, brown, long grain, 1 cup/195g	216	2	0
RICE, white, long grain, 1 cup/158g	205	0	0
ROLL, dinner, egg (2-1/2"/6cm diameter), 1 roll	107	2	1
ROLL, hamburger or hot dog, plain, 1 roll	120	2	0
SALAD DRESSING, French, commercial, 1 tbsp/16g	73	7	1
SALAD DRESSING, Italian, commercial, 1 tbsp/15g	43	4	1
SALAD DRESSING, vinegar & oil, homemade, 1 tbsp/16g	72	8	1
SALAMI, beef, cooked, 1 slice	68	6	3
SALMON, Atlantic, farmed, cooked in dry heat, 3 oz/85g	175	11	2
SARDINES, Atlantic, canned in oil, 1 cup/149g	310	17	2
SARDINES, Pacific, canned in tomato sauce, 1 cup/89g	165	9	2
SAUSAGE, blood, 1 slice	95	9	3
SAUSAGE, chorizo, pork & beef (4"/10cm link), 1 link	273	23	9
SCALLOPS, breaded & fried, 6 pcs	386	19	5
SHRIMP, breaded & fried, 3 oz/85g	206	10	2
SHRIMP, cooked in moist heat, 3 oz/85g	84	1	0
SNAP BEANS, green, boiled, 1 cup/125g	44	0	0
SOUP, chicken noodle, canned, chunky, ready to serve, 1 cup/240mL	91	2	1
SOUP, chicken rice, canned, chunky, ready to serve, 1 cup/240mL	127	3	1
SOUR CREAM, imitation, cultured, 2 tbsp/29g	60	6	5
SOYBEANS, boiled, 1 cup/172g	298	15	2
SPAGHETTI SQUASH, fresh, cubed, 1 cup/101g	31	1	0
SPINACH, boiled, 1 cup/180g	41	0	0
SPINACH, fresh, 1 cup/30g	7	0	0
STRAWBERRIES, fresh, halved, 1 cup/152g	49	0	0
SUCCOTASH, boiled, 1 cup/192g	221	2	0
SUNFLOWER SEEDS, dry roasted, w/ salt, 1 cup/128g	745	64	7

Sodium	Carbs	Fiber	Protein
(Milligrams)	(Grams)	(Grams)	(Grams)
13	39	5	8
45	4	2	1
18	131	6	5
1	15	8	1
10	45	4	5
2	45	1	4
191	18	1	3
206	21	1	4
134	2	0	0
243	2	0	0
0	0	0	0
296	0	0	3
52	0	0	19
752	0	0	37
368	1	0	19
170	0	0	4
741	1	0	14
919	38	0	16
292	10	0	18
190	0	0	18
1	10	4	2
840	10	1	8
888	13	1	12
29	2	0	1
2	17	10	29
17	7	0	1
126	7	4	5
24	1	1	1
2	12	3	1
33	47	9	10
525	31	12	25

Description of food	Calories	Fat	Saturated Fat
	(kcal)	(Grams)	(Grams)
SWEET POTATOES, cooked, baked in skin (5"/13cm long x 2"/5cm diameter), 1 potato	103	0	0
TANGERINE, fresh (2-1/4"/6cm diameter), 1 fruit	40	0	0
TOFU, fried, 1 pc	35	3	0
TOMATO, orange, fresh, 1 tomato	18	0	0
TOMATO SAUCE, canned, 1 cup/240mL	59	0	0
TROUT, cooked in dry heat, 3 oz/85g	162	7	1
TUNA, canned in oil, drained, 3 oz/85g	158	7	1
TUNA, canned in water, drained, 3 oz/85g	99	1	0
TURKEY BREAST, pre-basted, w/ skin, roasted, 1/2 breast	1089	30	8
TURKEY, fryer-roasters, breast, w/ skin, roasted, 1/2 breast	526	11	3
TURNIPS, fresh, 1 lg	51	0	0
WAFFLE, plain, homemade (7"/18cm diameter), 1	218	11	2
WATERMELON, fresh, diced, 1 cup/152g	46	0	0
WHITE BEANS, boiled, 1 cup/179g	249	1	0
WINE, all, 1 fl oz/30mL	24	0	0
WINTER SQUASH, all varieties, fresh, cubed, 1 cup/116g	39	0	0
YOGURT, fruit varieties, nonfat, 8 fl oz/240mL	233	0	0
YOGURT, plain, low fat, 8 fl oz/240mL	154	4	2
YOGURT, vanilla, low fat, 8 fl oz/240mL	208	3	2
ZUCCHINI, fresh, w/ skin, 1 cup/113g	19	0	0

Sodium	Carbs	Fiber	Protein
(Milligrams)	(Grams)	(Grams)	(Grams)
41	24	4	2
2	10	1	1
2	1	1	2
47	4	1	1
1284	13	4	3
57	0	0	23
337	0	0	23
287	0	0	22
3430	0	0	191
182	0	0	100
123	12	3	2
383	25	0	6
2	12	1	1
11	45	11	17
1	1	0	0
5	10	2	1
142	47	0	11
172	17	0	13
162	34	0	12
11	4	1	1

notes

notes

PETER PAUPER PRESS
Fine Books and Gifts Since 1928

Our Company

In 1928, at the age of twenty-two, Peter Beilenson began printing books on a small press in the basement of his parents' home in Larchmont, New York. Peter—and later, his wife, Edna—sought to create fine books that sold at "prices even a pauper could afford."

Today, still family owned and operated, Peter Pauper Press continues to honor our founders' legacy—and our customers' expectations—of beauty, quality, and value.

personal progress chart

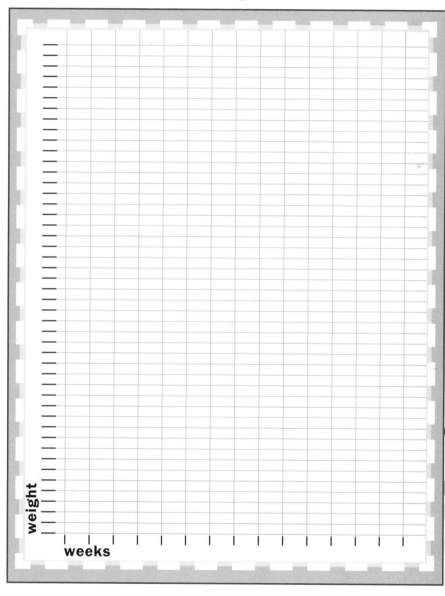